HOSPITALIST RECRUITMENT AND RETENTION

I enjoyed spending time with you this weekend.

HOSPITALIST RECRUITMENT AND RETENTION

Building a Hospital Medicine Program

Kenneth G. Simone
Hospitalist and Practice Solutions

WILEY-BLACKWELL

A JOHN WILEY & SONS, INC., PUBLICATION

Copyright © 2010 by Wiley-Blackwell. All rights reserved.

Wiley-Blackwell is an imprint of John Wiley & Sons. formed by the merger of Wiley's global Scientific, Technical and Medical business with Blackwell Publishing.

Published by John Wiley & Sons, Inc., Hoboken, New Jersey.
Published simultaneously in Canada.

No part of this publication may be reproduced, stored in a retrieval system, or transmitted in any form or by any means, electronic, mechanical, photocopying, recording, scanning, or otherwise, except as permitted under Section 107 or 108 of the 1976 United States Copyright Act, without either the prior written permission of the Publisher, or authorization through payment of the appropriate per-copy fee to the Copyright Clearance Center, Inc., 222 Rosewood Drive, Danvers, MA 01923, (978) 750-8400, fax (978) 750-4470, or on the web at www.copyright.com. Requests to the Publisher for permission should be addressed to the Permissions Department, John Wiley & Sons, Inc., 111 River Street, Hoboken, NJ 07030, (201) 748-6011, fax (201) 748-6008, or online at http://www.wiley.com/go/permission.

Limit of Liability/Disclaimer of Warranty: While the publisher and author have used their best efforts in preparing this book, they make no representations or warranties with respect to the accuracy or completeness of the contents of this book and specifically disclaim any implied warranties of merchantability or fitness for a particular purpose. No warranty may be created or extended by sales representatives or written sales materials. The advice and strategies contained herein may not be suitable for your situation. You should consult with a professional where appropriate. Neither the publisher nor author shall be liable for any loss of profit or any other commercial damages, including but not limited to special, incidental, consequential, or other damages.

For general information on our other products and services or for technical support, please contact our Customer Care Department within the United States at (800) 762-2974, outside the United States at (317) 572-3993 or fax (317) 572-4002.

Wiley also publishers its books in a variety of electronic formats. Some content that appears in print may not be available in electronic formats. For more information about Wiley products, visit our web site at www.wiley.com.

Library of Congress Cataloging-in-Publication Data:

Simone, Kenneth G.
    Hospitalist recruitment and retention : building a hospital medicine program / Kenneth G. Simone.
        p. ; cm.
    Includes index.
    ISBN 978-0-470-46078-8 (pbk.)
    1. Hospitalists. 2. Hospitals–Personnel management. I. Title.
    [DNLM: 1. Hospitalists–manpower.   2. Personnel Administration, Hospital–methods.
3. Personnel Selection–methods.   4. Personnel Turnover.   WX 203 S598h 2010]
    RA972.S553 2010
    362.11068–dc22
                                                                            2009043686

Printed in the United States of America

10 9 8 7 6 5 4 3 2 1

To Matthew and Olivia, with love

In loving memory of my brother Steve, forever in my heart

CONTENTS

PREFACE

Recruitment and retention of physicians in all specialties remains a national challenge. This challenge applies to both outpatient and inpatient physicians, primary care and specialist physicians, as well as private, government, and hospital-owned practices. As I've traveled across the country consulting with many hospitalist programs, it became apparent that recruitment and retention of physicians was a significant challenge for most programs, both old and new (and an Achilles heel for many). In my professional experience, practices and programs have encountered a vast array of recruitment and retention problems, resulting in destabilization of their hospitalist programs. These problems have included:

- *Inadequate planning.* Many programs fail to appropriately esti-mate the demand for their services (at the program's onset and over time) and thus fail to anticipate staffing requirements. In addition, many programs fail to plan and time the hiring of physi-cians (e.g., sequencing) when multiple providers are needed. They have failed to develop short- and long-term strategic staffing plans.
- *Lack of a clearly defined recruitment process.* Many hospitalist programs have failed to create a well-planned and choreographed recruitment process, leading to missed opportunities and/or a hiring mismatch. Physician recruitment is a buyer's market. This is par-ticularly true for hospitalists. It has been estimated that there are approximately 20,000 practicing hospitalists at the present time. The Society of Hospital Medicine (SHM) projects that there will be 30,000 hospitalists by 2010 and upward of 50,000 hospitalists by 2030 [1]. These numbers are phenomenal for a specialty just over a decade old. Yet, if you were to review the "hospitalist wanted" ads in medical journals, on the Internet, through direct mailings, or on the SHM Web site (to name a few sources), you would find that many hospitalist programs are recruiting for additional hospitalists. Factors accounting for this are explored in the book. Thus, pro-grams that do not clearly define the recruitment process, or those who fail to act promptly, may lose highly qualified candidates.

- *Hiring mismatch.* Many programs hire providers who do not fit in with the practice "culture." There is a mismatch between the vision, values, and objectives of the hospitalist program and the newly hired physician. This can lead to disruptive behaviors within the hospitalist practice, low morale, and can result in poor provider and program performance.
- *Lack of retention plan.* Many programs have been successful in finding a good physician–practice fit but failed in support and integration of the new physician into the practice, hospital, and community. A poorly developed retention plan or the absence of one can lead to physician turnover. Physician turnover can result in staff shortages, which may lead to program instability (e.g., be disruptive to the "chemistry" of a practice), provider job dissatisfaction, provider burnout, and subsequent poor clinical outcomes. Provider turnover can be quite costly to a hospitalist program, as numerous costs are associated with replacement of providers. These costs include those associated with recruitment (e.g., travel, lodging, sign-on bonuses, medical school loan repayment, relocation expenses, lost productivity for hospitalist and hospital staff during the recruitment process), headhunter fees, and revenues lost during provider shortages. In addition, programs may experience inappropriate ancillary utilization and an increase in the length of stay as a result of being understaffed, negating two of the major benefits of having a hospitalist program. This ultimately will decrease the return on investment for the subsidizing entity.

For startup hospitalist programs, development of an effective recruitment and retention plan at the onset will be invaluable in supporting a program's success. Too often, new hospitalist programs are derailed as a result of hiring the wrong physician (especially if it is the first hire). Whereas an established program will probably survive a poor recruitment choice, a new program, because of its lack of history within the medical community, may not have that luxury. Although there are no guarantees that a candidate will be the ideal hire, having a process in place will provide a foundation on which a program can make a choice objectively and effectively.

This book is designed to guide hospital administrators, hospitalist administrators, hospitalist clinical directors, medical staff leaders (chief medical officer, vice president of medical affairs, department chiefs), physician recruiters, hospitalist physician candidates, and physician practice managers through the recruitment and retention process. It analyzes current trends in hospitalist medicine and explores factors contributing to the challenges associated with recruitment and retention. These trends are supported by data from the latest SHM survey (2007–2008) which are incorporated throughout the book.

Tools and strategies that support the successful recruitment and retention of physicians are presented. To succeed at this challenging task it is vital that hospitalist program personnel understand the dynamics of recruitment and retention and acknowledge common pitfalls. Keep in mind that the creation of a recruitment and retention plan does not guarantee success. Meticulous preparation and flawless execution of a plan combined with an honest and transparent approach will go a long way to supporting the successful recruitment and retention of outstanding hospitalist physicians.

Acknowledgments

I would like to thank my wife, Julianne Simone, for her patience and assistance during this project. Her critical ear, constructive feedback, and creative suggestions were immensely helpful in the completion of this project. Without her this project could not have reached its full potential.

I would also like to thank Joseph Miller, senior vice president at the Society of Hospital Medicine, for providing assistance with the 2007–2008 SHM biannual survey. Joe remains a trusted and reliable confidant.

KENNETH G. SIMONE

1 Physician Supply and Demand

Physician supply and demand in many specialty fields affects hospitalist practice recruitment and retention significantly. There are several dynamics that affect the balance between physician supply and demand (see Exhibit 1.1). Some of these dynamics are universal to all physicians, whereas others are uniquely relevant to hospitalists. We explore these dynamics in this chapter.

1.1 THE AGING MEDICAL WORKFORCE

The existing physician workforce continues to age. This includes primary care as well as specialist providers. According to the American Medical Association (AMA) and reported by Cejka Search, 67% of practicing physicians are over the age of 42. Specifically, 18% are over the age of 61 and 49% are between 42 and 60. One in three male physicians and one in eight female physicians are over 55 years of age. As these physicians retire, there is a scarcity of replacement candidates. These candidates typically represent a new generation of doctors, accompanied by a very different set of residency experiences, professional expectations, and life goals (see Section 1.14).

Many disenfranchised physicians are either decreasing their clinical hours or retiring early, thereby compounding the aging workforce phenomenon. A survey conducted by the AMA and the Association of American Medical Colleges (AAMC) in 2007 [2] supported this observation. The survey indicated that 33% of physicians over the age of 50 would retire today if they could afford to do so. In a survey conducted in May and July 2008 by Merritt, Hawkins and Associates (for the Physicians' Foundation), 49% of physicians indicated that they planned either to reduce the number of patients they see or to stop practicing entirely within three years [3]. Forty-five percent of

Hospitalist Recruitment and Retention: Building a Hospital Medicine Program,
By Kenneth G. Simone
Copyright © 2010 Wiley-Blackwell

Exhibit 1.1   Physician Supply and Demand Dynamics

Physician supply and demand dynamics is one of the most significant factors influencing physician recruitment and retention. These dynamics include:

- Number of medical school graduates
- Number of residency programs and seats
- Number of international medical graduates
- Government policy
- Health of the U.S. economy
- Insurance industry
- Specialty choice
- Physician productivity
- Work schedules
- Number of full-time employees (FTEs)
- New medical technologies
- Aging physician population/retirement patterns
- Growing and aging patient population
- Utilization of nonphysician clinicians (NPCs)

physicians surveyed said they would retire today if they had the financial means.

Hospitalist providers can have a positive impact on both the aging and disenfranchised medical workforce. They can provide inpatient medical care for these physicians' patients. This may decrease the work burden and improve the lifestyle of these doctors, thus prolonging their careers. In effect, hospitalists can stretch the physician workforce, providing an immense benefit to the medical community as a whole.

1.2   THE GROWING AND AGING POPULATION

According to the U.S. Council on Graduate Medical Education (COGME), while the number of physicians will increase from 781,200 FTEs in 2000 to 971,800 in 2020 (a 24% increase), after 2015 the rate of the population growth will exceed the rate of physician growth [4]. The AAMC states that in the last 25 years the U.S. population has increased by 31%. The U.S. Census Bureau estimates that between

2005 and 2020 the projected population below 65 will grow 9% and the population 65 and older will grow by 50%!

This rapid increase in the aging population will be compounded in states such as Florida, West Virginia, Pennsylvania, Maine, and Iowa, which rank 1 to 5, respectively (according to the U.S. Census Bureau's 2007 census estimates) for the percent of the population who are over 65. Add North Dakota, South Dakota, and Rhode Island into the mix when one looks at the percent of the population over 85 years of age (although this population is much smaller) and the problem becomes greater. Include Vermont and New Hampshire as well when considering the oldest states by median age (see Exhibit 1.2). Keep in mind that

---

Exhibit 1.2 *Population Estimates by Age and Geography*

The following data are derived from 2007 U.S. Census Bureau population estimates classified by age and geography. These tables provide information on the aging population using various criteria.

Rank	Geographic Area in the United States	Percent
Percent of the population who are 65 years and over		
1	Florida	17
2	West Virginia	15.5
3	Pennsylvania	15.2
4	Maine	14.8
5	Iowa	14.7
Percent of the population who are 85 years and over		
1	{ Florida	2.7
	{ North Dakota	2.7
3	Iowa	2.6
4	South Dakota	2.5
5	{ Pennsylvania	2.4
	{ Rhode Island	2.4
Median age (in years) of the population		
1	Maine	41.6
2	Vermont	40.8
3	West Virginia	40.4
4	Florida	39.9
5	New Hampshire	39.8

healthcare utilization increases after 45 years of age. In addition, the elderly use many more services, representing a significant increase in healthcare dollars and demand for physician services. This will burden an already underserved workforce, as is evidenced by states with the greatest number of elderly patients.

1.3   DECREASED MEDICAL SCHOOL MATRICULATION

According to the AAMC, medical school applications declined in the United States for the first time between 1996 and 2002. This decline created a deficit in the physician recruitment pool that the medical profession has only recently come to realize. Additionally, between 1982 and 2001 the number of students enrolled in U.S. medical schools increased by 7% while the U.S. population grew by 23% [4]. This resulted in a 13% decrease in medical school students per capita. Current estimates indicate that the U.S. population will increase by 18% between 2000 and 2020, while medical school enrollment will increase by approximately 4%, leading to a further decline in medical students per capita. The effects of this decline are compounded further by the rapid rate of growth in the aging U.S. population.

The COGME, a national advisory body that makes policy recommendations regarding the adequacy of the supply and distribution of physicians, predicts that if current trends continue, demand for physicians will outweigh supply significantly by 2020. It recommends that medical schools expand the number of graduates by 3000 per year by 2015 [4]. The AMA recognizes this impending shortage and is recommending a 30% increase in the capacity of medical schools.

1.4   THE CHANGING DEMOGRAPHICS OF MEDICINE

The demographics of medical school graduates have changed dramatically in the last two decades (see Exhibit 1.3). According to the AAMC, the number of male applicants has decreased recently. Since 2003, medical school applications have increased, which coincides with the increasing number of women applying to medical school [5]. Additionally, the number of female and international graduates currently enrolled in U.S. medical schools has risen. For the first time in modern medicine, more women than men are graduating from medical school (54% of medical school graduates born after 1980 are women).

Exhibit 1.3   Gender-Related U.S. Physician Workforce Facts

Physician workforce demographics in the United States have changed considerably in the last several years. Women are playing an increasingly prominent role in the medical profession. These changes have significant implications on the physician workforce. The following is a sample of gender-related facts:

- One in three male and one in eight female physicians are over 55 years of age.
- One in four physicians is female.
- During the last three decades the proportion of new medical school graduates who are female has risen from 10% to close to 50%.
- Female physicians are 7% more likely to choose nonsurgical specialties.
- Female physicians spend fewer hours per year providing patient care.
- Female physicians are less likely to practice in rural areas.
- Female physicians tend to retire slightly earlier than do their male counterparts.

The AMA reports that women now make up approximately 50% of the U.S. medical resident pool. Female physicians typically seek practice opportunities that allow them to balance their professional and personal lives. Female physicians work approximately 18% fewer hours per week (0.8 FTE) than male physicians. This greatly reduces the overall number of physician hours available and the overall physician supply.

Although this trend may affect the physician workforce (in general) negatively, it may be something that hospitalist programs can capitalize on. Recruiting programs should consider if it's in a program's best interest to allow part-time physicians and/or job sharing. Hiring part-time physicians can provide a recruitment advantage for a program as well as increasing the staffing flexibility of the practice.

Programs considering recruitment of international medical school graduates (IMGs) should be aware of particular factors affecting the placement of these physicians. Many IMGs have geographic employment limitations, due to their visa status. For example, a J-1 visa requires that physicians return home to their country for two years after residency training unless they agree to practice in designated underserved areas for three years.

Historically, IMGs have been recruited to work in areas in which it is difficult to recruit, which are underserved, and which typically are rural. In many instances, when they fulfill their visa commitments, IMGs move on to other geographic locations (e.g., suburban or urban). This creates turnover and a potential physician shortage in these areas, which may already be experiencing recruitment challenges. Introduction of the H1-B visa has further compounded the problems in underserved areas. The H1-B visa does not require a physician to return home or work in an underserved area for three years. This has prompted many IMGs to work in suburban or urban locations that are not underserved. As a result, underserved areas are recruiting fewer IMGs.

1.5   THE COST OF MEDICAL SCHOOL AND THE GRADUATE DEBT BURDEN

The cost of medical school has contributed to the physician workforce shortage as well as to the recruitment and retention challenges faced by some practices. The following are examples of how the high cost of medical school and/or physician debt burden has affected the recruitment marketplace.

- Although there have been studies documenting that medical school is an excellent investment [6], high tuition cost has deterred potential applicants from applying. In a national survey conducted by the AAMC in 2004, students who appeared qualified for medical school were polled regarding why they didn't apply. Cost was a major prohibitive factor for all students and the leading factor for minority students (black, Hispanic, and Native American).
- The cost of medical school, accompanied by lost potential earnings (during the seven to 10 postcollege training years), has left many residency graduates seeking employment opportunities that provide immediate financial security rather than starting their own private practice. Many of these candidates sign on with the practice that offers the best financial package. These graduates may also be promised limited work hours, no hospital responsibilities, and minimal or no call as a lure. Additionally, they may not hesi-

tate to move on for a more lucrative offer in the future (which affects physician retention).

- Although this phenomenon does not change the absolute number of practicing physicians, it certainly has an effect on physician supply and patient access dynamics. Physicians with set work hours, limited call, and no hospital responsibilities will affect both the medical staff and local hospital (e.g., emergency department unassigned call, hospitalist program). It may also have a positive or negative effect on patient access in the community. These practices (e.g., hospital-owned practice, large national management company–owned practice) tend to have the financial resources to control the market. They may be clustered in suburban and urban areas, which may limit access for patients in the more rural areas (e.g., if physicians choose these practice opportunities over the rural sites).

- The debt burden may also be a motivational factor when these graduates choose a specialty. Primary care is considered an endangered species because so many medical students are going into specialty fields which provide a greater income stream throughout their career. Many medical school graduates are gravitating toward such fields as invasive radiology and interventional cardiology. As a result, numerous geographic areas in the United States are suffering from a shortage of primary care physicians, thus limiting healthcare access for many patients.

- Finally, the graduate debt burden may influence the practice location for many residency graduates. These doctors may choose geographic locations where insurance reimbursement is highest. Typically, these locations are in metropolitan areas with higher patient density. This may further the difficulties of rural recruitment.

Discussion of these financial factors should provide the reader with an understanding of the impact on both the workforce shortage and the current marketplace recruitment and retention dynamics. This information may also assist hospitalist programs when they create a recruitment package and/or develop their practice scope of service. For example, your program may decide to offer medical school loan repayment, a sign-on bonus, and a flexible schedule in order to compete in the marketplace and attract top candidates.

In addition, many underserved rural communities can only support one physician in a particular specialty. It would be virtually impossible to recruit this physician without practice support or backup. The physician would need to be available 24/7 (twenty-four hours a day/seven days a week) 365 days each year. Hospitalists can play a significant role in recruiting this specialist. They can provide hospital management for all of the specialist's patients as well as cover his or her emergency department night calls [similar to the services provided for primary care physicians (PCPs)]. Having this hospitalist support would allow these underserved areas to be successful in recruiting specialists into the community, benefiting the community, hospital, and hospitalist program.

1.6   THE CHANGING ROLE OF THE SPECIALIST

Traditionally, specialists have played a significant role in the active management of hospitalized patients. Over the last several years they have shifted their focus away from active management toward providing consultations (e.g., one-time evaluation of the patient) and performing procedures. This has placed an increased burden on other physicians, typically hospitalists, to assume the day-to-day management of these hospitalized patients. This specialist phenomenon may increase the burden on the already understaffed and overworked hospitalist provider. This may lead to decreased hospitalist job satisfaction, burnout, and provider turnover.

Several factors contribute to the changing role of the specialist.

- Over the years there have been great advances in medical technology (both diagnostic and therapeutic). This has shifted the training focus for many specialty residency programs away from direct patient care and toward interventional procedures. Graduating residents leave training programs eager to apply their skills and the latest technologies. With increasing specialist clinical expertise, both patient and physician expectations have changed accordingly.
- Another dynamic at play is the physician's financial incentive to perform procedures. The current U.S. healthcare payor system rewards procedure-oriented skills far greater than cognitive skills. For physicians coming out of training programs with large medical school debt and armed with a vast array of technical skills, the decision is easy.
- Finally, specialists who limit hospital privileges to consultations and procedures are typically excused from emergency department

(ED) unassigned call. This is a significant benefit, as many cases presenting to the ED are time consuming, offer little if any financial reward (many patients are uninsured), and may keep the physician in the hospital all night long. This can affect the provider's schedule and workload the following day, affect his or her quality of life, and affect job satisfaction negatively.

Many hospitalist programs have developed strategies to deal with this specialist phenomenon. Some have developed co-management protocols and services, particularly for both general and orthopedic surgery patients. These programs may increase their physician staffing ratios, hire NPCs to assist them, and create preprinted evidence-based order sheets to assist their hospitalist providers. If your program has done so, it is worthwhile to discuss this with potential candidates. It will illustrate that your program is progressive as well as supportive of the growing responsibilities that hospitalists are assuming. Knowing that a program is proactive and supportive of its staff will go a long way toward retaining these physicians.

1.7 THE CHANGING SCOPE OF PRIMARY CARE

The scope of primary care has been influenced by several dynamics in the last 10 to 15 years. The advent of managed care in the early 1990s made a significant impact on the role of primary care. Managed care referred to these physicians as gatekeepers and rewarded them for both the size of their patient panel (providers were paid a capitated fee per patient per month) and their ability to keep utilization and cost down. Many doctors responded by increasing their patient panel and availability to these patients. This required additional office hours, which made it difficult to sustain both an outpatient and inpatient practice and a family life. As a result, many physicians dedicated themselves to outpatient medicine and looked to colleagues in the medical community (e.g., doctors who were later coined *hospitalists*) to provide their patients with hospital care when needed.

The rapid growth in medical technological advances during this time was another major influence shaping the scope of primary care. These technological advances made it very difficult for any physician to stay current with all the diagnostic and therapeutic options available to patients. Failure to stay current could compromise patient care. It could also put the physician at increased medicolegal risk. Keep in mind: Patients who were admitted to the hospital were sicker and more complicated, necessitating a high acuity level of medical care. Thus, many primary care physicians felt that it was in the best of interest of their patients to be treated in the hospital by those doctors who regularly provide care for the critically ill. These hospital-dedicated physicians (hospitalists) were also more readily available to these patients.

The national focus on patient safety and quality initiatives has also influenced the practice of medicine (and primary care scope) in the twenty-first century. Hospital and physician performance regarding patient outcomes, morbidity and mortality, and medical errors are widely publicized and, therefore, transparent. Physician and hospital accountability have been brought to the forefront. Hospitals are turning to hospitalist programs to oversee these initiatives and to provide the bulk of the medical care in their institutions. Conversely, PCPs have focused their attention on developing outpatient quality assurance plans (e.g., diabetes and asthma registers) to address these initiatives and to demonstrate the quality of care they provide to patients. This has led to a renewed emphasis on specialization (e.g., inpatient and outpatient).

The clinical pressures that accompany the "jack of all trades and master of none" and the medicolegal risk to maintain competence is too great for some primary care providers. As a result, many established physicians have decreased their scope of practice, contributing to a relative decline in the physician workforce. For example, as more primary care physicians relinquish their hospital privileges, an increased burden will be placed on hospitalists to care for these patients. Also, these primary care physicians will no longer be available to provide hospital care for the uninsured (e.g., "unassigned" ED patients) as they did previously. Either the existing pool of hospitalists will need to increase their workload, or programs must recruit additional physicians.

This primary care trend decreases the relative number of physicians practicing inpatient medicine. This places more pressure on hospitalists, who will absorb these hospitalized patients as well as assume more unassigned ED calls. At the same time this trend also serves to support hospitalist medicine. These primary care providers are customers of the hospitalist practice. They serve as a large referral base from which a hospitalist program can grow its practice. Many programs view this PCP base as job security for their hospitalists. Your hospitalist program may consider the PCP–hospitalist relationship in this manner as well. When hospitalist candidates come to town for an interview, share this information with them. It is advantageous for the candidate to understand the extensive referral base and PCP support that your program enjoys.

1.8 THE AVAILABILITY AND ACCESSIBILITY OF TRAINING PROGRAMS

The availability of postgraduate training programs (e.g., the number of programs and the number of seats in each program) for various specialties can have an impact on the supply of physicians entering a specialty field. Furthermore, medical school indebtedness can have an effect on specialty preference and thus the number of applicants vying for a particular residency program (see Section 1.5). For example, in popular residency programs the number of applicants may be considerable, thus making entrance into that particular program and/or specialty field more difficult. This may have a domino effect on many medical fields, especially the primary care specialties. The number of practicing primary care physicians, in turn, will have an effect on the workload and scope of service for hospitalists.

1.9 TECHNOLOGICAL ADVANCES

Medical and technological advances can have a significant impact (negative or positive) on the demand for physician services. These advances can allow physicians to provide new services. For example, new protocols in cardiology recommend early intervention for patients with acute coronary syndrome. This increases the demand for invasive cardiologists. In addition, these invasive procedures may help prevent costly surgeries (i.e., coronary artery bypass graft), decreasing the demand for cardiothoracic services. To further this point, if these procedures result in increased life expectancy, this may translate into greater use of healthcare services over time (e.g., increase the demand for physician services).

In some cases pharmaceutical or diagnostic testing advances may provide a substitute for physician services. For example, the creation of a vaccine may decrease the disease burden of a particular illness (e.g., pneumonia, shingles, polio). Another example is the creation of immunomodulators. These agents treat a wide array of diseases, from AIDS to multiple sclerosis to rheumatoid arthritis, to name a few. Take rheumatoid arthritis, for example: Modulators help control this disease and prevent joint destruction, diminishing the need for orthopedic surgical intervention.

Diagnostic testing advances may also directly affect physician services. The evolution of computed tomography (CT) scan–assisted diagnostics such as cardiac CT scanning may eventually reduce the need for invasive cardiac diagnostics. Finally, technological advances such as gene therapy may prevent costly medical conditions and all of their sequelae, thus reducing the demand for certain services and expertise. Conversely, gene therapy may increase life expectancy, translating into greater use of healthcare services over time.

1.10 THE INCREASING REGULATORY RESPONSIBILITIES PLACED ON PHYSICIANS

The 2007 AAMC and AMA survey of physicians over age 50, mentioned earlier in the chapter indicated that older physicians cited increased regulation of medicine as the key factor influencing retirement plans. Historically, physicians over 50 years of age practiced in an era in which they had complete freedom to order diagnostic studies, prescribe medications, and admit their patients to the hospital. No pressure was placed on appropriate chart documentation or the need for utilization of preprinted evidence-based guidelines. "Pay-for-performance" was what occurred after a physician submitted a charge, "preexisting conditions" were what a physician considered when creating a diagnostic and therapeutic medical plan, and "prior authorization" was what a physician provided to his staff so that they could order various studies and/or medications.

In the "new world order" of healthcare, physicians have seen their professional autonomy shrink along with the reimbursements they receive for their services. They spend more time on administrative issues and second-guess paperwork. This paperwork involves completion of prior authorizations to justify the need for specifically prescribed medications and therapies. It may also involve completion of precertification paperwork to obtain approval from an insurer, allowing coverage for medically necessary diagnostic studies. In many instances, physicians must painstakingly document the presence of a preexisting condition before an insurer will even consider paying a physician for services rendered.

Direct patient care and access has been affected negatively by both voluminous paperwork and restrictive protocols. In the Physicians' Foundation survey cited earlier, 49% of physicians reported that the amount of time they devote to nonclinical paperwork has increased in the last three years. Furthermore, 63% of physicians said that nonclinical paperwork contributed to less time spent with their patients.

Physicians must also contend with increasing regulations placed on them in the form of federal mandates [e.g., the Centers for Medicare and Medicaid Services (CMS)] and national (e.g., the Joint Commission) initiatives, to name a few. For example, physicians are being "graded" based on clinical outcomes, treatment complications, and customer satisfaction. In the outpatient setting, doctors are responsible for creating chronic disease registers (e.g., diabetes, asthma), and reporting quality performance indicators. In the inpatient setting, a physician's performance is measured by adherence to core measures, evidence-based clinical guidelines, and pay-for-performance indicators. The latest CMS initiative has Medicare denying payments to hospitals for "never events," which are defined as preventable errors, injuries, and infections that occurred while the patient was in the hospital. This Medicare "do not pay" initiative will certainly change the way that physicians practice hospital medicine.

Over the years, various governing agencies (e.g., licensure boards and specialty boards) and credentialing entities (e.g., hospital medical staff credentials committee, managed care and preferred provider organizations) have increased the number of physician requirements needed to maintain and demonstrate current competency. These requirements may include attending "live" continuing medical education (CME) programs, accumulating a set number of CME hours per year, and sitting for board recertification testing every seven to 10 years (for some specialties). These activities involve time, money, and paperwork, all pulling physicians away from their medical practice.

Although many of the initiatives presented above are worthy and necessary (e.g., quality and patient safety initiatives), some have proved onerous and others unnecessary to many physicians. A number of doctors feel disenfranchised. They have been heard to say things like "I didn't sign up for this. I went to medical school to treat patients!" Consequently, many physicians are leaving the medical profession at an earlier age. This occurrence has contributed to the physician shortage.

The hospitalist movement has flourished in the aftermath of these restrictions. In many ways, hospitalists are the answer to the perceived problems created by these regulations. In response, hospitalists have embraced quality care and patient safety initiatives, electronic medical records (EMRs), evidence-based clinical guidelines, the Joint Commission's core measures, and Medicare's pay-for-performance program, to name a few. Many hospitalist programs have created policies, procedures, and protocols to deal with these regulations and initiatives. When recruiting it would be worthwhile to take the time and share what your hospitalist program has done to address these issues and put your program on the cutting edge.

1.11   RISING PRACTICE EXPENSES AND DIMINISHING RETURNS FROM THE INSURANCE INDUSTRY

Annually, the balance of practice expenses vs. income is a challenge for all physicians. This is especially true for office-based physicians such as family practitioners (FPs), internists, and pediatricians. Consider the following: The average FP has a 55 to 60% total expense ratio! The *total expense ratio* is defined as total practice expenses, including staff salaries, office and medical supplies, rent/mortgage, and so on, divided by total collections. This means that the average FP has less than 45% of his or her earnings available *before* taxes. This expense ratio is significantly greater than for procedure- or hospital-oriented specialties such as surgery and anesthesiology. These specialties provide the majority of their services in the hospital. Their need for both office staff and space is greatly reduced compared with the primary care specialties. Thus, hospital-based specialists have comparatively lower operating costs than those of office-based physicians.

According to William F. Jessee, president and CEO of the Medical Group Management Association (MGMA), primary care physician practice costs and overhead continue to rise at "staggering rates." On average, physician practice expenses increase by approximately 5 to 6% each year. This is a result of rising wages and benefits for office staff, higher salary packages for providers (e.g., base salary, sign-on bonus, loan repayment, moving expense, etc.), as well as higher costs for both office overhead and malpractice coverage. The rise in practice overhead is compounded by the fact that the insurance reimbursement that physicians receive does not match the inflationary rates to run an office. In a recent survey, only 17% of doctors believed that the financial status of their practice was "healthy and profitable" [3].

The annual impending Medicare and Medicaid cuts magnify this problem further. In the Physicians' Foundation study, 82% of physicians stated that their practices would be "unsustainable" if these Medicare cuts were made. Additionally, 65% of physicians reported that Medicaid reimbursement was less then their cost to provide medical services.

Physician practice management is becoming more complicated due to the financial pressures and dynamics listed above. Nearly half of all physicians spend one full day per week managing their business, which results in less time spent with patients [3]. (This diversion from patients is exacerbated by the voluminous paperwork associated with insurance companies.) In many cases, physicians are faced with difficult decisions regarding office staffing. Personnel costs account on average for about one-fourth of the operating costs of internal medicine practices. Thus, some practices address rising overhead expense by laying off valuable staff. This can affect both staff and practice efficiency negatively and disrupt office dynamics. As a result of these financial pressures, many physicians are leaving medical practice earlier in their careers.

Hospitalist programs may find it useful to target these struggling physicians. Inpatient management of their patients by the hospitalist program would free time at the beginning and end of the workday, allowing these doctors to be more efficient (working in one venue) and see more patients, thus improving their bottom line. Develop a marketing plan to assist your program in this endeavor. Share this plan would potential candidates. This will convey the fact that your hospitalist program is aggressive in establishing and maintaining market share. This addresses both program stability and job security for the potential hire.

1.12   UTILIZATION OF NONPHYSICIAN CLINICIANS

With the rising costs associated with running a physician practice, non-physician clinicians (NPCs: advance practice nurses, physician assistants) offer a cost-effective option for many primary care and specialty practices. There are significant financial savings (e.g., recruitment, salary, malpractice) when an NPC is employed rather than a physician. Utilization of these providers has grown considerably as more physicians (and patients) became comfortable with their level of expertise. It is not surprising that the nonphysician workforce continues to grow.

The decision of a practice to employ an NPC implies certain responsibilities. Physician assistants (PAs) require direct physician supervision, whereas advanced practice nurses (APNs) may practice independently (only as an outpatient provider) in many states (varies from state to state). For those practices employing one or both of these professionals, physicians must dedicate a significant amount of time and resources to advancing the training and skills of these providers. In certain circumstances, NPCs are trained to perform procedures.

The utilization of NPCs has had both a negative impact on physician demand and a positive impact on physician supply. For example, if an APN establishes an independent practice in a community, this may decrease the demand for physician services (e.g., competing interests). On the other hand, if the APN (or PA) joins a physician practice, this may allow the physician to become more efficient and thus more productive (e.g., see more patients), increasing the relative supply of physician services. Having NPCs available in a practice may also translate into fewer physicians needed in the practice to provide care (e.g., decreasing physician demand).

The use of NPCs within hospitalist programs is increasing. They are utilized in a variety of ways, depending on the program. Their utilization is discussed in detail in Chapter 11. If your hospitalist program employs NPCs, it is helpful to share this with the candidate during the recruitment process and discuss the program's use of these practitioners. The candidate should be queried about his or her familiarity and comfort with the utilization of these healthcare professionals.

1.13   GOVERNMENT POLICY

The U.S. government continues to have a profound impact on the supply and demand of physicians and the specialty they choose. This impact can occur through federal regulations as well as payment policies (e.g., Flexner Report, Bane Report, the Health Education Facilities Act, Emergency Health Personnel Act). For example, the government can increase or decrease funding for medical school education (e.g., National Institute of General Medical Sciences, National Institutes of Health, Title VII Health Professions Education Programs) and residency training (Medicare subsidy). The following serve as specific examples:

- In the recent past, the U.S. government capped the number of residents and fellows eligible for Medicare reimbursement. This had a negative impact on physician supply because it discouraged teaching hospitals from increasing the number of residents it trained. This policy was made at a time when there were fears of a physician surplus.
- Title VII of the Public Heath Service Act includes a government program encouraging physicians to practice medicine in rural and underserved areas. The intent of the program is to increase physi-

cian access for those persons living in rural and traditionally underserved geographic locations. This program has affected the distribution of physicians and thus its relative supply in these areas.

- The Accreditation Council for Graduate Medical Education (ACGME) created a Resident Work Hour Regulation in 2003 which limited the number of hours worked by residents in a week (averaged over four weeks). This policy drastically reduced the relative physician workforce (e.g., supply) by decreasing hospital "house staff" work hours in teaching hospitals. This affected residency faculty as well by increasing their work hours each year on the hospital wards (reducing their availability for research and classroom teaching). As a consequence, many teaching programs hired hospitalists to cover these hours, resulting in a greater demand for physician (e.g., hospitalist) services.

- In December 2008, the Institute of Medicine (IOM) released a report (which was requested by Congress in 2007) recommending new restrictions on medical resident's duty hours and workloads. One of the major changes suggested was that shifts not exceed 16 continuous hours. In addition, the resident must receive a five-hour "protected sleep period" between 10 in the evening and 8 in the morning. Other proposed recommendations include an increase in the number of days that residents have off each month, moonlighting restrictions during resident's off hours, and setting a four-night maximum for in-hospital night shifts (with 48 hours off after three or four consecutive nights). If these recommendations are accepted, this will further stress the physician workforce and is likely lead to increased involvement of hospitalist physicians in teaching hospitals.

Government policy can also affect physician supply and demand by both regulating the number of seats available in medical schools and by regulating the number of IMGs entering the country. The government can further affect physician supply and demand in specific specialties by addressing the differential payments for healthcare services. This has an impact on training opportunities and specialty choices. Specialists (especially procedure-focused doctors) make significantly more money than primary care physicians, due to the current reimbursement model that rewards procedural work over cognitive work. This disparity has had a negative effect on the number of physicians going into primary care in the United States.

1.14 GENERATIONAL EXPECTATIONS

There are significant differences between the mature, baby boomer, gen X, and millennial generations. These differences result from the varied experiences that each generation has had on a personal level as well as on a global level. On a personal level, for example, the baby boomers typically grew up with stay-at-home moms, whereas gen X'ers typically had dual working parents (e.g., both worked outside the home). On a global level, the mature generation grew up during the Great Depression and World War II, boomers during both the Cold War and the start of the Viet Nam war, gen X'ers during the Viet Nam war and Watergate, and millennials during the technological explosion. As a consequence, there is considerable divergence in how each generation views its world. This perception, in turn, affects individual values, goals, and expectations both personally and professionally. These generational differences have had a significant impact on physician supply and demand dynamics.

It will be extremely valuable for recruiting programs to familiarize themselves with different generational perspectives in order to develop strategies and tools for successful recruitment and retention of these physicians. Having perspective on the candidate's motivations, values, and expectations will provide your program with a recruitment advantage. It will also support long-term retention of these physicians.

According to the AMA in a brief review of physician workforce demographics:

- Sixty-seven percent of practicing physicians fall into the mature and boomer generations (e.g., 42 years of age and over); 88% are male.
- Approximately 33% of practicing physicians represent the gen X sector (27 to 41 years of age); 58% are male and 42% are female.
- Millennials (people born after 1980) are just now emerging from medical school. Although small in numbers, currently 54% are women.

One can gather several inferences from these data; the majority of physicians currently in the workforce are middle-aged males, the number of women entering medicine is increasing significantly, and the gen X and millennial generations will soon lead the medical workforce. Refer to Exhibit 1.4 for an outline of the generational differences.

Exhibit 1.4   Generational Differences

The following are characteristics usually attributed to each generation. Although these generational classifications refer to an era and thus a specific period of time, a person may be identified by his or her values and actions rather than by the year in which he or she was born.

- *Mature (a.k.a. silent or GI or peacemaker) generation*
  ○ Born approximately 1923–1943
  ○ Raised during the Great Depression and World War II
  ○ Social conservatism
  ○ Firm leaders who believe in teamwork
  ○ Committed and disciplined
  ○ Loyal and willing to sacrifice
  ○ Empty nesters with growing amounts of leisure time
  ○ First generation of woman to move into the workforce in great numbers
  ○ Strong human relations skills
  ○ Involved in cultural and societal issues
- *Baby boomer generation*
  ○ Born approximately 1946–1964
  ○ Raised during post–World War II economic boom
  ○ Respect authority and work hard out of loyalty
  ○ Value and expect long-term job placement
  ○ Pay dues; self-sacrifice is a virtue
  ○ Willing to work long hours
  ○ High expectations
  ○ Like being in control of their environment
  ○ Value creativity and adventure
  ○ Independent workers
  ○ Ideologically passionate
- *Generation X (a.k.a. gen X or MTV generation)*
  ○ Born approximately 1965–1980
  ○ Raised during the Viet Nam war and Watergate
  ○ First generation in which both parents probably worked outside the home
  ○ Paying dues is not relevant

- Question authority
- Cynical and detached, leading to self-reliance
- Place high value on relationships
- Appreciate organizations that provide strong orientation and mentoring programs
- Work–life balance; value personal time and job flexibility
- Independent lifestyle; divorce twice as prevalent for children in this generation and therefore they value family, friends, and other personal interests
- Distrust of institutions and less loyalty to employers than previous generations; witnessed parents getting laid off for their loyalty to an organization; therefore, their first loyalty is to themselves
- Change jobs frequently; focused on developing portable skills they can market to enhance their future career success (and move from one employment situation to another)
- Entrepreneurial, do-it-yourself attitude
- Less involved in politics and public policy

- *Millennial (a.k.a. generation Y or echo boomer) generation*
  - Born approximately 1980–2000
  - Raised at the end of the Cold War
  - Parental involvement and structured activities in which "Nobody wins unless everybody wins"
  - More conventional, favor large institutions
  - Respect authority and follow the rules
  - Bright, driven, technologically savvy; subject to greater academic pressures than previous generations
  - Work well within structure; team-oriented, enjoy collaboration and cooperation
  - Need constant feedback and workplace recognition
  - Optimistic and respond well to humor and truth
  - Attracted to the potential for lucrative positions and long-term job security
  - Seek "perfect" work–life balance; unwilling to work as long hours as prior generations have
  - Socially conscious; value family, religious faith, honesty, and integrity

An understanding of the motivational factors guiding the physician recruitment pool will allow your program to focus on candidates having similar values and objectives. It will also enable you to concentrate your recruitment and retention efforts on those areas that appeal to the particular candidate. The following examples will illustrate this point.

- The survey by the AMA and AAMC mentioned earlier indicated that 66% of doctors under 50 (e.g., boomers, gen X'ers, Millennials) were not interested in working longer hours for more money. In addition, 71% of young doctors identified having family and personal time as an important factor in a desirable practice. Hospitalist programs offering a flexible schedule and blocks of time off may have a recruitment advantage. If your program has had difficulty with retention, evaluate your program model and schedule. Making adjustments in these areas may significantly improve your ability to retain physicians (and recruit new doctors). In Chapter 5 we discuss practice models and scheduling in detail.

- According to the *Journal of the American Medical Association* (JAMA), three recurrent characterizations of gen X physicians are a desire for flexible schedules, a preference for the latest technology, and cynicism about organizations. Each of these areas has particular implications for recruitment and retention. Practice opportunities that appeal to gen X physicians will emphasize the organization's mission and vision for the future, use the Web, stress the availability of flexible schedules (including job sharing and part-time positions), and be sensitive to the call schedule burden. Developing a solid orientation and mentorship program for these new physicians will go a long way toward retention.

- Cam Marston, author of the book *Motivating the "What's in It for Me" Workforce*, reports that gen X'ers and millennials guard their time carefully. These people are principled, loyal to their families, but less loyal to their employers than more previous generations. Rather than viewing a practice opportunity as the start of a long-term commitment, they may see it as a means for building "a personal—and portable—portfolio of career assets" [7]. It may be said that physicians born in the gen X and millennial eras view medicine as a profession and not as a calling or lifestyle. Building a hospitalist practice that instills trust and teamwork (e.g., camaraderie) may provide these people with the security they need to commit long term to your program.

Tip: Early in the recruitment process, assess the values and motivations of the candidate. Focusing on the priorities and concerns of each candidate during the interview may provide your program with a strategic advantage. For example, if your program offers well-defined work hours and no call duties, these should be stated clearly. If the program permits job sharing or part-time work, present this to those candidates seeking flexibility. If your program offers internal moonlighting opportunities, this should be shared with those physicians looking to maximize their income. These are just a few examples of the types of information that your program should consider sharing with physician candidates. One word of warning: Never sell a candidate a false bill of goods.

After reviewing the dynamics affecting the U.S. physician workforce, it is no surprise that the medical profession is bracing for an impending physician shortage in the near future. The face of medicine as we know it today will most certainly change in the next several years. Hospitalists are positioned to emerge as the leaders in this new model of healthcare. They may stabilize the workforce by improving quality of life translating into professional satisfaction. This, in turn, may delay retirement for some physicians and aid in recruitment and/or retention of physicians within the community. This will have the overall effect of stretching the physician workforce. Keep in mind that your hospitalist program must develop internal systems that support these professionals.

2 The Hospitalist Marketplace

To further understand the forces at play in hospitalist recruitment and retention, a review of the hospitalist workforce is necessary. In this chapter we explore the characteristics of practicing hospitalists, their work responsibilities, and the characteristics of hospitalist medicine groups as a whole. Knowledge of the intricacies of other hospitalist programs (the competition) will be valuable and provide your program with an objective measuring stick to gauge the competitiveness of your employment opportunity.

The data presented were taken from the Society of Hospitalist Medicine (SHM) biennial survey in 2007–2008 (with comparisons to the 2005–2006 survey shown in parentheses). These data were collected from October through December 2007. Although there are other sources of hospitalist data in the literature (e.g., the Medical Group Management Association), SHM's data are widely recognized as *the source* describing the current hospitalist landscape (from a program and provider perspective). These data should provide valuable information as long as the reader is aware that there are limitations to any survey based on the methodology employed.

2.1   AGE, GENDER, AND YEARS EMPLOYED AS A HOSPITALIST

Mean age
   Physician leaders: 43 years old (42)
   Nonleaders: 39 years old (38)

The survey data indicated that hospitalist leaders are older than nonleaders, which makes sense from a maturity and work experience perspective. Typically, hospitalist leaders have considerable work

Hospitalist Recruitment and Retention: Building a Hospital Medicine Program,
By Kenneth G. Simone
Copyright © 2010 Wiley-Blackwell

experience in the field before they're hired for a leadership position. Additionally, the survey indicated that internal medicine- and pediatric-trained subspecialists are older than the average hospitalist. This may be associated with the number of postgraduate training years required to complete subspecialty training. This observation may also indicate that these subspecialists were previously established in a private (or hospital-owned) practice and transitioned later in their career to a hospitalist position. This transition may be for financial (e.g., a more lucrative hospitalist position) and/or lifestyle purposes. It may also represent the physician's dissatisfaction dealing with the administrative side of the medical profession. Query those physicians transitioning from a traditional practice into a hospitalist practice during the interview to ascertain why they are making a change.

From this latest SHM survey, the mean hospitalist was born during the gen X era, which has several implications regarding hospitalist program recruitment and retention strategies. Possessing knowledge of this fact will provide your program with valuable information with which to approach the perspective candidates. The specific gen X characteristics were discussed in Chapter 1. It would be worthwhile to review these characteristics and focus your recruitment efforts accordingly.

Gender
    Male: 65% (65%)
    Female: 35% (35%)

Leadership by gender
    Leaders: male 80% (80%); female 20% (20%)
    Nonleaders: male 63% (62%); females 37% (38%)

Both the total number of male hospitalists and the number of male hospitalist leaders are significantly higher than the number of female hospitalists. This is not unexpected when comparing the total number of males and females currently practicing medicine in the United States. In the future, these ratios may change as the number of females entering medical school is on the rise. The increase in female physicians translates into potential growth in the number of female hospitalists. Hospitalist medicine may be very attractive to the female physician workforce because it provides flexibility. This flexibility may not be available in other practice venues or specialties.

Conversely, the number of female hospitalist leaders may be less likely to increase, due to the relative inflexibility of these leadership positions. Nationally, hospitalist program leaders tend to be full-time employees who spend at least 50% of their time or more (typically, 80%) providing clinical care. Although they spend more time doing nonclinical work than their nonleader counterparts, hospitalist leaders have approximately the same number of patient encounters per year [8]. As stated in Chapter 1, female physicians typically work 18% fewer hours per week than their male counterparts, which would make it difficult to direct a hospitalist program clinically.

Mean years employed as a hospitalist
    Leaders: 6.7 years (5.8)
    Nonleaders: 3.7 years (3.1)

Mean years employed by current practice
    Leaders: 5.1 years (4.7)
    Nonleaders: 3.0 years (2.8)

Analysis of the survey data indicates that hospitalist leaders have more hospitalist work experience than do nonleaders. Hospitalist leaders within a given program are also employed longer. These findings are not surprising, as many programs look for leaders possessing significant hospitalist experience. Additionally, programs may look within their own practice to fill the leadership position when an opening arises. Thus, leaders tend to have a longer tenure with one practice than do nonleaders. Finally, being a hospitalist program leader may lend itself to greater workplace stability (for the leader), resulting in greater workplace retention. When there are no internal candidates for the leadership position, the recruitment team may consider physicians who have extensive work experience in one hospitalist practice. Workplace longevity typically reflects both professional (and personal) stability and professional competence.

Many hospitalist programs have run into difficulties when their leader was either inexperienced as a program director or lacked sufficient experience in the trenches prior to rising to the role of practice leader. "Battlefield" experience is a wonderful teacher, as it exposes the physician to various clinical situations in addition to operational and administrative challenges. This experiential phenomenon does not differ from professions where successful leaders must be adept in all areas of their business. Having said that, if your program opts for an inexperienced candidate, surround this person with experienced physician leaders and/or mentors from the medical community.

2.2 HOSPITALIST EDUCATION

Percent graduates of U.S. medical schools
    Leaders: 85% (85%)
    Nonleaders: 71% (72%)

Hospitalist training
    General internal medicine: 82.3% (78%)
    Internal medicine subspecialty: 4% (4%)
    Internal medicine–pediatrics: 3.1% (3%)
    General pediatrics: 6.5% (11%)
    Family medicine: 3.7% (3%)

Currently, the majority of hospitalists are trained in internal medicine. This is understandable as most internal medicine residents spend most of their training in hospitals. Consequently, these physicians are most comfortable practicing in a hospital setting.

As the demand for hospitalists outpaces the supply, a new pool of hospitalists must emerge from other specialties. FPs may be a natural fit based on their residency training. These physicians are taught to treat the entire person and to coordinate all aspects of a patient's care. Many FPs have considerable clinical experience treating patients in the hospital as well as in the outpatient setting. These doctors can relate to their customer base (e.g., referring PCPs) by possessing an understanding of the multitude of PCP responsibilities as well as possessing knowledge of the resources available in the community for their patients at discharge. They can also be called upon to provide pediatric hospital services if the need arises.

Physicians trained in internal medicine–pediatric (IM-Ped) are also a good option for hospitalist program staffing. In this instance, recruiting programs must be sensitive to the fact that most IM-Ped physicians expect to have a minimum number of adult *and* pediatric cases, to maintain current competency in each field. This is particularly true for pediatric cases, where the average daily census (ADC) is typically lower than for adults.

The role of NPCs in hospitalist programs is expanding to stretch the workforce further. Programs that employ NPCs successfully have a structure in place that provides for appropriate support and supervision of these providers. For this model to succeed physicians within the practice must buy into the NPC concept.

In the future, many internal medicine, family medicine, and internal medicine–pediatric residency training programs will provide a hospitalist tract and/or fellowship program, thereby grooming these new physicians to be the hospitalists of the future. Until then, the future supply of hospitalists will come from the existing physician workforce. Many established practitioners who are currently in private practice have grown intolerant of the increasing regulations placed on them with little to no financial reward. Many other physicians are tiring of the business and administrative pressures associated with private practice. For some doctors, hospitalist medicine may make more sense than retiring from medicine prematurely.

Now that the reader has a better understanding of the qualities of hospitalists, we will explore the hospitalist marketplace, examining characteristics of hospitalist medicine groups (e.g., the competition).

2.3   HOSPITALIST PRACTICE LOCATION

By region
  East: 31% (24%)
  South: 28% (26%)
  West: 21% (22%)
  Midwest: 20% (27%)

By surrounding community
  Small urban (less than 1 million): 48% (49%)
  Large urban (greater than 1 million): 31% (33%)
  Rural: 21% (18%)

There was a significant increase in the number of survey respondents from the East and a significant drop in the number from the Midwestern region of the country, possibly indicating the growth of hospitalist programs in the eastern United States. The survey broke these regions down further into nine census regions (New England, Mid-Atlantic, East North Central, West North Central, South Atlantic, East South Central, West South Central, Mountain, and Pacific). Refer to Exhibit 2.1 for a definition of states by geographic region. When these data were analyzed, the South Atlantic had the greatest distribution of responding programs, possibly indicating the location of the greatest concentration of hospitalist programs. The Mountain region represented the smallest concentration of programs. The largest percent variation by census region from the 2005–2006 survey to the 2007–2008 survey was experienced by New England (plus 4%), East North Central (minus 4%), and Mountain (minus 4%) regions.

Exhibit 2.1   SHM Geographic Census Regions

The following are the geographic regions used in the SHM 2007–2008 biennual survey:

- East: ME, VT, NH, MA, CT, RI, PA, NY, NJ, DC, DE, MD
- South: VA, WV, NC, SC, TN, KY, GA, FL, AL, MS, LA, TX, AR
- Midwest: OH, IN, IL, MI, WI, MN, IA, MO, NE, KS, SD, ND, OK
- West: CO, UT, NM, WY, MT, ID, AZ, NV, OR, CA, WA, HI, AK
- New England: ME, VT, NH, MA, RI, CT
- Mid-Atlantic: NY, NJ, PA
- East North Central: OH, IL, WI, IN, MI
- West North Central: IA, MO, MN, KS, NE, SD, ND
- South Atlantic: DE, MD, DC, WV, VA, NC, SC, GA, FL
- East South Central: KY, AL, TN, MS
- West South Central: LA, AR, OK, TX
- Mountain: CO, UT, NM, WY, AZ, NV, MT, ID
- Pacific: CA, OR, WA, AK, HI

When the data were evaluated by population size, the greatest variation in practice growth from the 2005–2006 survey to the 2007–2008 survey was experienced by rural hospitalist programs (plus 3%). These rural areas tended to have hospitalist programs in hospitals with fewer than 100 beds (66%). Additionally, more rural hospitalist programs were treating adults and children (41%), and were newer (32%). These findings are not surprising because rural areas tend to have smaller hospitals.

Rural hospitals typically have challenges recruiting and retaining physicians in all specialties, due to factors described in Chapter 1. As a result, many rural hospitals have strategically recruited primary care physicians (i.e., FPs) and NPCs, who can provide a wide variety of services for the medical community. They can provide adult and pediatric services for hospitalized patients, thus alleviating the need to recruit a greater number of providers, which could prove problematic. Finally, the high percentage of new rural hospitalist programs may indicate that the hospitalist model of medical care is being embraced by these smaller hospitals to meet the medical needs (and combat the physician shortage) in their respective communities.

Small urban area hospitalist groups, on the other hand, were associated with significantly fewer hospitals with 100 or fewer beds compared to rural areas (27% vs. 66%, respectively). Hospitalist programs in these areas were affiliated more with hospital-only groups and management companies (59%) than with major teaching programs (36%). Conversely, more large urban area hospitalist groups were affiliated with hospitals having 500 or more beds (56%) and more were affiliated with academic institutions (48%). These programs tended to be more established, as only 18% were less than one year old.

A review of the practice location provides information regarding potential sources of candidates for your program. It also allows your program to target hospitalist candidates in specific locations based on their professional experiences (e.g., bed size, patient demographics, teaching experience) and living preferences (e.g., geographic location, population size, climate). In other words, recruitment efforts can be directed at hospitalist candidates based specifically on clinical exposure and location if desired. Focused searches may improve the prospect of hiring and retaining a hospitalist candidate who is compatible with your program.

2.4 HOSPITALIST EMPLOYMENT MODEL AND HOSPITAL TEACHING STATUS

Employment model
>   Hospital: 40% (34%)
>   Academic institution: 24% (20%)
>   Local hospitalist only: 14% (12%)
>   Multispecialty/PCP medical group: 11% (14%)
>   Management company: 8% (19%)

Teaching status
>   Nonteaching: 43% (48%)
>   Major teaching (e.g., member of the Association of American Medical Colleges or Council of Teaching Hospitals): 28% (28%)
>   Other teaching: 28% (25%)

Analysis of the current data indicates that the majority of hospitalist programs are either owned or subsidized by hospitals. This is not surprising considering the significant amount of subsidy needed to support a successful hospitalist program. It is particularly true for programs providing added-value services, as most of these activities are not reimbursable by insurance companies. Many private hospitalist groups cannot provide the funding required to run a thriving program without a subsidy from an outside source (i.e., a hospital). According to the 2007–2008 SHM biennual Survey, the mean financial support (from sponsoring hospitals) per FTE physician was $97,375. The survey also indicated that 91% of all hospital medicine groups receive a subsidy (the mean amount received was $949,410). Hospital subsidy is the logical choice since it is the hospital that benefits directly from these services.

Successful recruitment and retention strategies for hospital-run programs should include aligning the candidate's vision and values with those of the institution and community. Too often, a physician is hired who does not buy into the program or the concept that his or her job responsibilities include serving the mission and objectives of the sponsoring hospital. The candidate should have a clear understanding of who his or her employer is.

Successful recruitment and retention strategies for local hospitalist-only groups include screening and identifying candidates who possess an entrepreneurial spirit. Physicians in private practice must have a keen business sense to maximize income and survive in the competitive marketplace. Private hospitalist practices are at a financial disadvantage compared to hospital-owned practices (who typically have large cash reserves to subsidize the program). Private groups compensate for the lack of large cash reserves by maximizing their productivity. This may result in a large patient census per provider and long work hours.

Finally, the candidate should be screened regarding geographical and lifestyle preferences before being brought to town. These hospital-run programs tend to be located in hospitals with fewer than 100 beds, and more were located in rural areas. Rural living has its advantages and disadvantages both in terms of the practice of medicine and the standard of living for the candidate and his or her family.

The increase in market share for academic hospitalist programs is not surprising, for a few reasons. The restrictions placed on the number of hours a resident can work in an average week (by the ACGME) placed greater demands on the residency faculty to service these uncovered hours. These additional hours spent on the hospital wards took faculty away from their research (and from the classroom in some instances). This contributed to work dissatisfaction for many faculty, making it difficult for some residency teaching programs to retain these people. Consequently, many residencies created hospitalist programs to provide coverage on the hospital wards in response to the relative decrease in personnel. Some programs also utilize their hospitalist service to teach residents.

Recruitment and retention strategies for teaching hospitalist programs will differ from those for nonteaching hospitalist programs. The ideal candidate must enjoy spending time instructing interns and residents, teaching, and working in larger institutions. These hospitalists may also enjoy performing clinical research. They must be willing to live in suburban or urban geographical areas. Many academic hospitalist opportunities also involve government hospitals (50%), which may be a recruitment factor pro or con for some candidates.

2.5   CONTROL/HOSPITAL GOVERNANCE OF AFFILIATED HOSPITAL

Hospitalist hospital governance
    Not for profit: 12% (10%)
    For profit: 5% (3%)

The majority of hospitalist programs are associated with not-for-profit hospitals. Hospital governance may or may not have bearing on hospitalist recruitment and retention. In all likelihood there are greater financial pressures placed on hospitalist programs (and providers) subsidized by for-profit institutions. For example, greater emphasis may be placed on provider and program performance measures such as average length of stay (ALOS), cost per case, average daily census (ADC), and productivity [relative value units (RVUs)] in for-profit hospitals. These hospitals must be focused on the bottom line if they are to survive and stay in business. As a result, some providers may be uncomfortable working in such an environment.

2.6   HOSPITAL SIZE

Bed size
    501 or more: 24% (24%)
    201–300: 19% (20%)
    101–200: 19% (19%)
    301–400: 17% (16%)
    401–500: 11% (12%)
    100 or less: 10% (9%)

Earlier in the chapter we noted that many hospitalist programs associated with smaller hospitals (100 or fewer beds) are located in rural areas, and that many programs associated with hospitals of more than 500 beds are located in suburban or urban areas. Additionally, programs associated with these smaller hospitals tend to care for both pediatric and adult patients, whereas some programs associated with larger hospitals tend to be affiliated with academic institutions. The reader should be aware that these statements are generalizations and do not apply to all communities or to all hospitals. The take-home message is that the recruiting hospitalist program must clearly state the specific characteristics of their program, the characteristics of the sponsoring hospital, and the characteristics of the local community. This is explored in detail in Chapter 9.

Bed size can be a deciding factor for hospitalist candidates seeking employment. Consider that the number of beds and medical staff size in rural hospitals are typically smaller than in suburban communities. There may be fewer specialists and less backup for hospitalist providers in the smaller hospitals. Night call frequency may be greater than in large hospitals, due to a smaller pool of physicians with which to share the call. Medical resources and technology are usually limited in these rural areas. As a result, the hospitalist physician may be viewed as the go-to person, and the responsibilities and expectations placed on them may be quite high.

Smaller hospitals also tend to have a quaint feeling to them. Many employees know each other and many live in the same community. Frequently, physicians run into their patients when off duty, while grocery shopping, dining, or attending a play. The candidate must be made aware of this small town atmosphere before they are brought to town for an interview and before they are hired.

Hospitalist programs that are located in suburban or urban areas tend to be affiliated with larger hospitals (i.e., more beds). These institutions have a much different feel from their rural counterparts. They have a large number of physicians on the medical staff, and typically there are more specialists to provide backup to the hospitalist when the need arises. Night call frequency may be decreased compared to a rural program because there may be more physicians to share the call burden. The technology available at these hospitals may be on the cutting edge. The patient base may be more diversified and the number of patients cared for (i.e., daily census) significantly higher than in rural programs. The practice pace may be hectic and the expectations high from both hospital administration and the community at large. Hospitalist responsibilities may also differ from those of rural programs. The responsibilities may decrease because there are more resources from which the hospital can draw. Conversely, they may increase because there are more initiatives in a larger institution.

The communities in which these larger hospitals are located differ in characteristics from those in rural areas. Typically, there are more social, cultural, educational, and spiritual resources available to the candidate and his or her family. In addition, the spouse may have more employment opportunities available. In most cases, the physician can have relative anonymity when off duty. Recruiting program personnel must do their best to present the selling points that accompany the practice opportunity.

2.7   HOSPITALIST STAFFING

Mean number of staff
    Physician: 12.03 (8.81)
    Physician assistant: 0.6 (0.4)
    Nurse practitioner: 0.57 (0.43)
    Other clinical staff (i.e., RNs and case managers): 0.35 (0.26)
    Nonclinical staff: 1.59 (1.09)

Mean number of FTEs
    Physician: 9.75 (7.97)
    Physician assistant: 0.57 (0.32)
    Nurse practitioner: 0.43 (0.37)
    Other clinical staff (i.e., RNs and case managers): 0.27 (0.28)
    Nonclinical staff: 1.21 (0.89)

The mean number of physician staff, NPC staff, and FTEs has increased since the last survey. Specifically, the mean number of hospitalists was 49% higher for major teaching hospitals than for nonteaching institutions, and 66% higher in large urban areas than in rural areas. Additionally, physician staffing at adult-only hospitalist programs was 59% higher than at pediatric-only programs. Finally, staffing for hospital-owned hospitalist programs was 13% lower than the overall average.

The overall increase in hospitalist staffing may be reflective of the increasing nonclinical responsibilities assumed by today's hospitalists. In this scenario, staff growth has no relationship to (an increase in) the ADC of the program. Staff growth may also be explained in part by the increasing popularity of the hospitalist movement. In this case, more providers are referring their patients to the hospital to be cared for by hospitalists (i.e., an increase in the ADC of the program). Finally, the staffing increase may reflect an expansion of the program's clinical services, such as with programs offering co-management of surgical patients, 24/7 in-house coverage, code blue, and/or rapid-response team coverage.

When one analyzes staffing growth by hospitalist program characteristics, for-profit, pediatric, and hospitalist programs more than five years old had lower growth rates. Hospitalist programs less than one year old, those affiliated with government hospitals, those affiliated with major teaching programs, and those owned by a management company had higher growth rates. This makes sense since younger programs are in a growth mode and government and major teaching programs must fill the void left by resident work-hour limitations.

Hospitalist staffing data provide information on the hospitalist marketplace relating to both physician and program support. It also provides general information on staff size and the composition of the clinical staff. This information can be used for comparison purposes during recruitment, although staffing numbers without utilization data (e.g., annual number of admissions, consultations and encounters, average daily census) may be of limited value.

2.8 COVERAGE SCHEDULE AND NIGHT CALL RESPONSIBILITY

Coverage schedule
    Shift only: 48% (40%)
    Call only: 17% (25%)
    Hybrid: 35% (35%)

Night coverage
    On-site providers: 53% (51%)
    On-call from home: 27% (41%)
    Combination on-site and on-call: 16% (did not ask in the previous
        survey)
    No night coverage responsibility: 3% (8%)

Mean percentage of time working nights
    Nocturnists: 89%
    Nonnocturnists: 17%

An understanding of the coverage and night call schedules that hospitalist programs utilize will benefit your program. It will provide an idea of what type of schedule candidates are currently utilizing and what type of schedule they are seeking. Shift-only coverage schedules have increased in popularity in the last two years, while call-only schedules have decreased. This development is consistent with younger physicians' desire to attain work–life balance. Analysis of the survey indicates hospitalist management companies and hospital-employed practices were utilizing the shift-only model more than other hospitalist medicine groups. Conversely, pediatric hospitalist groups, mixed pediatric/adult hospitalist groups, and hospitalist practices affiliated with government hospitals and academic institutions utilized the call-only schedule more often.

It may be hypothesized that employment of a shift-only coverage schedule requires more physicians on staff than a call-only model. For example, in a call-only model the on-call physician works multiple shifts in a 24-hour period. In a shift-only model the same physician works only one shift; thus, more physicians are required to work in the same 24-hour period. To illustrate this point, if a program requires two physicians to work the day shift and one physician to work at night, in a call-only model two providers are needed (one day physician takes calls at night), while in the shift-only model three physicians are needed (two on days and a third physician to work the night shift). Utilization of more physicians in a practice translates into greater expense and, potentially, higher levels of subsidy needed to run the program. This could explain why large hospitalist management companies and hospital-employed groups can afford to utilize such a model. These groups typically have the financial resources that allow them to recruit a greater number of hospitalists.

Pediatric and academic hospitalist groups tend to have lower productivity (e.g., care for fewer patients) than hospitalist management companies or hospital-employed groups. Additionally, mixed pediatric/adult programs tend to be located in rural areas, where the hospitals are smaller and the referral base limited. It may follow that these groups have less capital available to hire a sufficient number of providers to allow for a shift-based practice model.

Regarding night call responsibilities, on-site coverage was utilized more by hospital-employed programs. This may be attributed to the hospital's desire to provide night coverage for the rapid-response team and code blue team by hospitalist physicians. In-house coverage by hospitalists may also provide relief for emergency department providers as well as provide support for the nursing staff. Although on-site night coverage is more expensive than "call from home," the hospital would benefit in many ways, thus providing a positive return on their investment. In contrast, call from home was utilized more by government hospitals, hospitals with fewer than 100 beds, and pediatric hospitalist groups. One may postulate that these programs may have a small number of hospitalists in their practice, which would make it difficult to dedicate a physician each night in the hospital.

2.9 HOSPITALIST PROGRAM GROWTH AND TURNOVER

Mean number of FTEs
Current: 11.18 (8.6)
One year ago: 8.99 (6.67)
Mean growth in FTEs over one year: 31% (29%)
Median number of staff leaving: 9% from 2005–2006 SHM biennual survey (there was no data set from the latest survey)

The latest SHM data indicate that hospitalist programs continue to expand. Hospitalist programs with the highest growth rates were new programs (less than one year old), programs associated with government hospitals, hospitalist management companies, and programs affiliated with major teaching hospitals. Growth of academic hospitalist programs is consistent with the fact that fewer resident work hours are available to cover the hospital wards, due to the Resident Work Hour Regulation of 2003 (see Section 1.13).

The latest SHM survey did not address program turnover (although the society recently completed a "focused survey" which was not available at the time of this writing). Data from the 2005–2006 SHM survey indicated that there was significant physician turnover (e.g., 9%) among the respondents. There are a number of reasons for this turnover (see Exhibit 8.2). This underscores the importance of developing effective retention strategies within your program.

3 The Role of the Hospitalist

Hospitalist medicine is the fastest-growing medical field in U.S. history. As stated earlier, there are approximately 20,000 hospitalists practicing in the United States at the current time, with estimates of 10,000 more by 2010. It would be an understatement to say that both the medical profession and healthcare industry have entrusted the future of hospital-based care to hospitalists. There are many reasons for this dramatic hospitalist growth. In Chapter 1 we discussed in detail factors affecting physician supply and demand.

In addition to physician demand–supply dynamics, hospitalist pro-liferation may be attributed to other factors. By virtue of their training and clinical experience, hospitalists bring a wide variety of skill sets to the table. Hospitalists excel in direct patient care, interacting with family units, working with other healthcare professionals, and function-ing within integrated healthcare delivery systems. Most hospitalists possess excellent communication skills and interact well with key stake-holders in the medical community. In addition, many excel in admin-istrative and leadership roles. Consider the fact that hospitalists have an appreciation for the financial aspects of medicine along with an understanding of the drivers of healthcare and one can see why these physicians are entrusted with such vast responsibilities.

Hospitalists are charged with improving patient care, patient safety, and patient access to the healthcare industry (including indigent popu-lations) while decreasing the cost of medical care (through a decreased ALOS and cost per case). They are also expected to improve both PCP job satisfaction and lifestyle in addition to the bottom line. Some hos-pitalists support teaching institutions by serving as residency faculty and/or providing coverage for residency teaching programs. Hospitalists also provide leadership within their respective institutions. Many hos-pitalists are called upon to provide leadership on a national level. With all these responsibilities and expectations placed on them, it is no

Hospitalist Recruitment and Retention: Building a Hospital Medicine Program,
By Kenneth G. Simone
Copyright © 2010 Wiley-Blackwell

wonder that hospitalists feel immense pressures from a multitude of sources. Hospitalist programs must be aware of these pressures affecting physician recruitment, job satisfaction, and retention.

Although hospitalists bring many things to the table, they will have a difficult time succeeding without practice support. Most hospitalist candidates are aware of this fact and search for programs providing such support. During recruitment, discuss the operational systems within your practice that support provider success. Those programs that do so improve their prospects of recruiting and retaining exceptional candidates. This is explored in greater detail in Chapter 9.

The following data describe the clinical and nonclinical activities of a typical hospitalist. They are derived from the 2007–2008 SHM survey with comparison to the 2005–2006 survey in parentheses.

3.1 HOSPITALIST PROGRAM PATIENT TYPE AND ENCOUNTER TYPE

Patient type
> Adult: 86% (79%)
> Children: 10% (15%)
> Adult and children: 4% (6%)

Encounter type
> Admissions, follow-ups, discharges: 73.6% (77.3%)
> Consultations: 8.2% (8%)
> Observation status: 8% (6.2%)
> Critical care: 4% (4%)
> Procedures: 2% (1.7%)

The majority of hospitalist programs care exclusively for adult patients. This is particularly true for both multistate hospitalist groups (i.e., national management companies) and local hospitalist groups as contrasted with academic or government programs. When the data were ratcheted down for pediatric-only hospitalist groups, the academic programs far outnumbered the other types of hospitalist programs (e.g., local groups, national management companies). Finally, the mixed adult and pediatric hospitalist groups tended to be in hospitals with fewer than 100 beds. These smaller hospitals (and hospitalist programs) are typically located in small suburban or rural areas. The existence of mixed adult and pediatric programs would make sense in these areas, as it would be very difficult to subsidize and/or staff separate adult and pediatric programs. These rural programs are generally staffed with NPCs and/or FPs. Many of the physicians in these programs are foreign graduates, for the reasons discussed in Chapter 1.

Most of the work performed by hospitalists is traditional inpatient medical care (e.g., admission, follow-up, and discharge of hospitalized patients). Some programs offer additional services, such as:

- Medical consultation
- Surgical co-management
- Pre- and postoperative care
- Procedure-oriented services (e.g., placement of central lines and Swan Ganz catheters, treadmill exercise testing, bedside cardiac ultrasound, thoracentesis)
- Palliative care
- Code blue and/or rapid-response team coverage
- Observation bed management
- Long-term acute care management

Gaining an understanding of a candidate's skills and interests will be advantageous for both the recruiting program and the candidate. For example, your program may decide to expand the services offered based on these skill sets. Conversely, if the candidate possesses procedural skills and interests that your program does not offer (e.g., bronchoscopy, colonoscopy), hiring this person may be a mismatch.

Hospitalist programs offering a vast array of clinical services may have a recruitment advantage or disadvantage, depending on how it's presented to the candidate. For example, clinical diversity provides many opportunities and challenges for physicians. It may present the opportunity to learn new clinical and administrative skills, and contribute to the growth and development of the physician as a professional. It may also represent additional job security for the hospitalist physician if the services are deemed indispensible to the hospital. Conversely, programs offering multiple services may be at a disadvantage if the candidate perceives these services as additional responsibilities (creating extra work for the physician).

The evolution of a hospitalist program should always be presented to the candidate, to illustrate the overall direction, progress, and vision of the program. Describe the objectives for each service, stressing how it provides value to both the program and the sponsoring hospital. A brief history of why a new service was created may help put things in perspective.

Discuss the staffing requirements, clinical and administrative responsibilities, policies, and procedures associated with each service. In addition, describe how these services interface with traditional hospitalist responsibilities (e.g., providing medical care for patients admitted directly to the hospitalist practice), discuss if the physician can choose specific services based on his or her interests (e.g., perioperative care, palliative care), and discuss how these duties affect the physician's work schedule. For example, if your practice offers rapid-response team coverage, provide the candidate with a detailed description of the hospitalist program's responsibilities. This includes discussing the rapid-response team's policies, procedures, and protocols, role of the hospitalist (e.g., team leader), hours of hospitalist coverage (e.g., daytime, nighttime, 24/7), and the composition of the team (e.g., nurse, respiratory therapy or intravenous infusion specialist).

3.2 HOSPITALIST TIME SPENT ON NONCLINICAL ACTIVITIES

Mean: 8.6% (11.6%)

In the last several years hospitalists have become an indispensable resource for both the medical staff and hospital in which they work. The role they play in the hospital has expanded beyond the delivery of direct patient care. This is not a surprise considering the perspective and skill set hospitalists bring to the table.

Hospitalist programs differ in the expectations they have for their hospitalist providers. Following are some examples of nonclinical duties (sometimes referred to as *added-value services*) in which hospitalists may participate. They may:

- Serve in medical staff leadership roles (e.g., president or chief of the medical staff, chief of internal medicine, family medicine, or pediatrics, quality assurance director)
- Serve in an educational role (e.g., with medical students, residents, nurses)
- Participate in research
- Participate on key medical staff committees (e.g., utilization management, pharmacy and therapeutics, quality/performance improvement, patient safety)

- Serve as the medical staff liaison to the information system department (i.e., for electronic medical records)
- Create and assist in the implementation of evidence-based clinical guidelines and patient safety initiatives
- Address compliance issues and performance measures

These nonclinical expectations are broad based and vary from program to program. Some of these responsibilities require the hospitalist candidate to possess strong business, time management, leadership, and interpersonal skills. Participation in these activities may provide the candidate with an opportunity to grow and build his or her administrative and leadership skills. This point should be stressed to the physician when discussing these nonclinical activities. If your program allows physician participation at CME courses pertaining to physician and/or medical staff leadership, inform the candidate.

Make no mistake: Hospitalist candidates look at the additional responsibilities they will assume if they sign on with your program. These responsibilities must be stated clearly at the onset of the recruitment process as well as in the job description. Be very clear about the support provided to the physician to accomplish the program's goals. If additional pay is associated with these nonclinical responsibilities, it would be beneficial to state that up front. The specifics of the recruitment process are discussed in Chapter 9.

3.3   LEADER TIME SPENT ON ADMINISTRATIVE ACTIVITIES

Mean: 29.5% (25%)

Hospitalist program leaders (i.e., clinical directors) have a wide variety of administrative responsibilities in addition to their clinical responsibilities. The specific expectations for the clinical director vary depending on the program. Over the last several years, the amount of time spent on administrative activities has increased for the director. What differs from program to program is how the director's administrative time is allocated and how he or she is compensated for this additional work.

The clinical and administrative responsibilities of the hospitalist clinical director should be defined clearly. This will support successful recruitment and retention of these personnel. All expectations should be stated in the job description and reviewed with the candidate during the recruitment process. Also, time management for administrative duties should be discussed. Some programs provide their clinical director with dedicated administrative time (i.e., time allotted during the workday or a specific day dedicated to these responsibilities). This dedicated block of time allows the director to change gears and focus on systems and programs needing attention. Although this strategy supports director success, many programs do not have the resources to allow such dedicated administrative time.

3.4   HOSPITALIST ACTIVITIES BASED ON LOCATION

The hospitalist marketplace was described in Chapter 2 by geographic location, teaching status, employment model, hospital size, and hospital governance (among other characteristics). In many ways, these characteristics drive the activities offered by the hospitalist program at these institutions. If your program is considering an established hospitalist candidate, be aware of the type of program from which he or she is coming. The candidate may possess various strengths or weaknesses based on the clinical experience and exposure.

The discussion that follows illustrates the skill sets that a candidate may or may not possess based on clinical experience. Be aware that broad generalizations are presented for the reader's consideration, to illustrate the point that all hospitalists do not possess the same clinical experience.

Critical Access Hospitals

Hospitalists working in critical access hospitals are charged with stabilizing patients within three days and either discharging them or transferring them to another institution. These physicians do not manage complicated patients with multiple problems requiring an extended stay in the hospital. Additionally, the hospitalist's exposure to critically ill patients may be limited, as frequently these patients are transported from the field to facilities capable of managing both the patient's acute illness and their extended needs (thereby passing the local critical access hospital). For example, the critical access hospitalist's experience with acute myocardial infarction (due to the new standard of acute intervention) and chronic ventilator patients may be limited.

Although critical access hospitalists may have limited clinical exposure and opportunity in some respects, they have a wide range of responsibilities placed on them because of their small medical staff size and limited resources. In addition, the number of hospitalist providers is often smaller, placing greater responsibility on these physicians. As a result, these hospitalists must possess excellent triage skills, must work well independently, and must be able to multitask.

Community Hospitals

Hospitalists working in community hospitals are usually exposed to a wide variety of clinical experiences. Depending on the size of the hospital, standard of care in the community, and medical staff support that these hospitalists receive, they may manage a wide variety of cases. On the other hand, they may not manage critically ill patients requiring tertiary care services (e.g., dialysis, open heart surgery), depending on the resources within the hospital and within the community. In many hospitals the community hospitalist serves as a jack of all trades for the medical staff.

Community hospital programs allow the hospitalist to build professional relationships with a variety of people, due to the smaller and more intimate size of a community hospital (compared to major medical centers). For example, hospitalists work collaboratively with the referring primary care groups, specialists, nursing staff, and case management department. They may even have the opportunity to assist in building the integrated healthcare delivery team. In this regard, these physicians may build their communication and leadership skills.

Major Medical Centers

Hospitalists at major medical centers are exposed to a wide variety of pathology and clinical challenges (e.g., a wide breath of experience). In many instances these medical centers serve as the referral center for outlying hospitals within a radius of several hundred miles. The hospitalist program may be expected to admit most (if not all) of these patients at the time of transfer. The hospitalists typically enjoy clinical support from many different specialties. This support may be a double-edged sword, depending on the rules of engagement with these specialists. For instance, it may be mandatory for the hospitalists to obtain a consultation from a specialist in specific situations (potentially limiting both the hospitalist's clinical involvement and his or her professional challenge). In addition, the intensive care unit may be closed (e.g., open only to intensivists). On the other hand, hospitalists at these major medical centers have access to a wide variety of clinical expertise as a result of specialist availability. This support may improve clinical outcomes in complex cases and expose the hospitalists to cutting-edge technologies.

In many instances, major medical centers have residency training programs in various specialty fields, potentially affecting the role of the hospitalist (and clinical experience) in the institution. The training programs may free hospitalists from providing code blue and rapid-response team coverage as well as from providing unassigned emergency department coverage. Hospitals with training programs may also expose hospitalists to teaching.

University Hospitals

Hospitalists working in university hospitals are exposed to a wide variety of clinical experiences, including residency teaching programs. The hospitalists may serve as residency faculty (in a hospitalist residency track or in a traditional internal medicine, family medicine, pediatric, or medicine–pediatric program), may provide coverage for the residency program, and may be involved in clinical research. They may also have limited contact with the residents if the hospitalist program does not interface with residents. The hospitalist's clinical experiences typically mirror those of hospitalists in major medical centers.

Long-Term Acute Care Facilities

Hospitalists working in long-term acute care facilities possess solid geriatric skills. They must manage acute exacerbations of chronic illnesses as well as chronic diseases requiring longitudinal care. Generally, these hospitalists work closely with nurses, therapists (e.g., physical therapy, occupational therapy, speech therapy, respiratory therapy), case management, social service, and the patient families. They must also be comfortable working in the rehabilitation and physical medicine milieu.

4 The Hospitalist Recruitment Pool

The lifeline for any successful hospitalist program, new or established, is the quality of its physicians. A physician of outstanding quality can be defined in many ways. Quality can refer to depth of clinical knowledge, breath of clinical skills, or can be based on clinical performance (e.g., clinical outcomes, complication rates, morbidity and mortality). Quality may also imply that a physician is compassionate, possesses outstanding communication skills, demonstrates good citizenship, or is flexible. Quality may also refer to a doctor's leadership ability, ability to teach, or ability to practice medicine in a fiscally responsible manner. Whatever your definition, all programs seek highly qualified physicians for their practice. It therefore benefits your hospitalist program to have an extensive recruitment network in place that gains you access to a wide variety of candidates. Access to a diverse pool of candidates enables your program to choose the appropriate physician based on the specific needs of the practice.

4.1 BUILDING YOUR RECRUITMENT NETWORK

Most hospitalist programs recruit on a continuing basis either because they are in a growth mode or are replacing a provider. The latest SHM survey indicated that the mean growth rate in FTE hospitalists was 31% in the last year! This implies that your program faces formidable recruitment competition. When building your recruitment network, familiarize yourself with the diverse candidate sources that are available. The hospitalist recruitment pool is extensive, and having these sources available will help the recruitment process move swiftly. It has been estimated that it can take between nine and 12 months on average to recruit a physician into a practice. A list of candidates can be created by utilizing a number of sources, as outlined in Exhibit 4.1.

Hospitalist Recruitment and Retention: Building a Hospital Medicine Program,
By Kenneth G. Simone
Copyright © 2010 Wiley-Blackwell

Exhibit 4.1 Candidate Sources

Early in the recruitment process your program must decide the extent of the candidate search (e.g., local, regional, or national). Based on this decision, a list of candidates can be created by utilizing any of the following resources:

- Advertising
  - Medical journals
  - Job Web sites (e.g., SHM Web site)
- Direct mailing to physicians
- Exhibiting and/or networking at medical conventions
- Hospital-employed recruiters
- Medical job fairs
- Networking with the medical staff and within the local community
- Networking with residency training programs
- Networking with state and local medical associations
- Networking with national medical societies (e.g., SHM)
- Personal referrals
- Recruitment agencies (contingent and/or retained)

Advertising

Placing an advertisement in medical journals is a traditional recruitment tool. If your program decides to utilize this tool, you must determine in which journals to advertise. This will help preselect your audience. For example, choosing *The Hospitalist* or *Today's Hospitalist* will focus your ad on hospitalists, whereas choosing *The Journal of the American Medical Association (JAMA)* will broaden your program's exposure to physicians in other specialty fields. If you decide to focus your search on a specific specialty (e.g., internal medicine, family medicine, pediatrics) consider placing an advertisement in the journal published by the respective specialty (and other journals associated with the specific specialty). It will be worthwhile to peruse various journals to gain an appreciation of the advertisement layout for each journal and to become familiar with your competition. These ads will also provide ideas on how you would like to differentiate your program from others.

Journal advertising is virtually effortless. It allows your hospitalist opportunity to be viewed by many readers and is one of the least invasive modes of recruitment for potential candidates. However, the effectiveness of journal advertising may be limited according to various sources in the literature, especially with the development of Internet advertising.

Physician recruitment via the Internet has become very popular. There are numerous recruitment Web sites (some are hospitalist specific), and many post both help wanted (e.g., employer) and job wanted (employee) ads. This provides exposure for both buyers and sellers in the hospitalist marketplace. SHM serves as an excellent online recruitment source for hospitalist programs and hospitalist physicians (www.hospitalmedicine.org/careercenter). Additional Internet job sites include (but are not limited to) PhyJob.com, PracticeLink.com, HOSPITALISTcareer.com, PhysEmp.com, and HospitalistJobs.com. It would be worthwhile to browse these sites, reviewing the job listings and hospitalist program advertisement descriptions.

In the late 1990s many residency programs utilized the Internet and some developed chat rooms to recruit residents to their programs [9]. It may be prudent for hospitals and hospitalist programs to proceed in a similar manner. It is now quite common for hospitalist programs to have their own Web site and links to attract potential candidates. Utilization of Web site development as a recruitment tool is discussed later.

Direct Physician Mailing

Direct physician mailing is a simple, yet limited tool to attract physician candidates to your program. As with journal advertising, the time and effort needed to complete this task is minimal. Mailing may now refer to the Postal Service and/or the Internet. Recruiting programs must either procure a mailing list for potential candidates or utilize a recruitment firm to provide this service. Mailings generate queries that may lead to new recruitment opportunities. If you utilize a recruitment firm for this task, keep in mind that they control access to the mailing list and will use the same lists for multiple clients. The overall yield for this particular strategy remains low.

Medical Conventions

Medical conventions provide an excellent forum to meet potential candidates either through a program exhibit booth or through networking. The operative term for this tool is *meet*. Networking and exhibiting imply a face-to-face meeting with physicians. This makes for a more personal approach to recruitment. This allows you to discuss your program in detail (geared toward the physician's questions and interests) and allows the candidate ample opportunity to provide both professional and personal information. During this encounter, assess your interest in the candidate as well as the candidate's interest in the opportunity and the likelihood that he or she will join the practice.

The recruitment opportunity may vary depending on the conference type and geographic location. Local and regional conventions (e.g., state society meetings, hospitalist chapter meetings, CME offerings) may increase your prospects of recruiting a physician successfully. Many physicians exploring employment opportunities (particularly those with families) prefer to stay in the same geographic region. However, this is not always the case. For those physicians willing to relocate to a different geographic area, networking at the annual SHM meeting provides great value and opportunity. It also provides your program with exposure to a national pool of candidates. The annual meetings for the American College of Physicians (ACP), the American Academy of Family Physicians (AAFP), and the American Academy of Pediatricians (AAP) may also represent opportunities to recruit for your program.

Medical Job Fairs

Job fairs are similar to medical conventions in that the recruitment opportunity allows for a face-to-face meeting between your program and the potential candidate. They differ from conventions in a few ways. For example, physicians at job fairs are specifically looking at job opportunities as opposed to conventions, society meetings, and CME events, where they are in attendance primarily for other purposes. Second, job fairs are typically attended by both residents and newly graduated physicians, whereas attendance at medical conventions consists primarily of physicians currently in practice. Established physicians searching for a job usually do not attend job fairs; rather, they carry out their search confidentially, often using a headhunter (so as not to undermine their current position).

Be aware of one potential drawback with job fairs. Unless it is a hospitalist-sponsored event, many of the physicians in attendance will be looking at opportunities in other specialties (e.g., they may not be hospitalists). Thus, your exposure to hospitalist candidates may be limited by using this recruitment modality. If you have access to residents as well as a local SHM hospitalist chapter in your community, consider coordinating a job fair through this organization.

Networking with Residency Training Programs

Networking with residency programs provides access to a continuous stream of potential candidates before they make their postgraduate decision. Hospitalist programs should seriously consider establishing and maintaining a relationship with residency programs. This relationship can be formal, such as committing to regular intern and resident clinical rotations on your hospitalist service (e.g., monthly or quarterly). It may also entail a formal commitment by your program to provide lectures to the residents. Either way, it will expose residents to your program and allow you access to these future doctors. If residents rotate on your service, it will allow you to evaluate their clinical acumen as well.

Recruitment Agencies

Recruitment agencies are frequently utilized by practices in all medical specialties. A variety of companies provide this service. Some are local or regional and others are nationally based. Before committing your program it is prudent to research each agency regarding both their placement success and their experience recruiting hospitalist physicians. In addition, discuss the financial arrangements before signing an agreement. Some agencies work on a contingent basis, whereas others require a retainer. There are variations for both of these arrangements which will either increase or decrease your financial exposure.

If your program elects to go with a recruitment agency, establish a close working relationship with them from the onset. The agency must have intimate knowledge of your program and employment opportunity. This includes information about the program's history, objectives, infrastructure, and operations. They must also be familiar with your program's staffing (support and clinical), practice model, and call schedule. Recruitment and retention success will be influenced by the agency's ability to present your program in a candid and appealing manner. It will be very costly and inefficient to bring a candidate to town on false pretenses.

Networking with the Medical Staff and Personal Referrals

Referrals from the medical staff or local medical community are excellent sources for candidates. These candidates are typically established within the medical community, and their endorsement should be considered strongly by the recruiting hospitalist program. Familiarity and trust with the hospitalist physician can translate into a larger market share for your program, particularly if the program is new and/or if there are competing hospitalist programs within the community. Presumably, from a lifestyle and personal perspective, the candidate (and his or her family) enjoys the community and geographic location since they're looking to stay in the region. Family and lifestyle considerations contribute to physician retention. This is discussed in greater detail in Chapters 8 and 9.

There are a few potential drawbacks to consider with local physician candidates. If the candidate is not viewed widely as an excellent physician, hiring this doctor may have a negative impact on your referral base. This is also true if there are unforeseen politics between this physician and your referral base. An additional question to ask is: Why is the physician leaving his or her current practice? Finally, if the physician is leaving an established practice, your program must be sensitive to the impact that this may have on that practice. The take-home message is that your program must perform its due diligence and proceed as you would with any candidate. That is, this candidate should go through the recruitment process your program has established.

Hospital-Employed Recruiters

Some hospitalist programs have the luxury of utilizing in-house recruiters who are usually hospital employed. This recruiter has intimate knowledge and personal experience working within the hospital, community, and presumably with your practice. Access to the recruiter is greater with an in-house presence, as is your ability to customize the recruitment approach. The cost and financial risk for these services may be more cost-effective than using a recruitment agency would be, depending on the specific relationship your program enjoys with the sponsoring hospital.

4.2   IDENTIFYING YOUR CANDIDATE POOL

Potential candidates may be found in competing hospitalist practices, established private (e.g., nonhospitalist) practices, or residency programs. These candidates may hail from a variety of fields as well (see Exhibit 4.2). According to the 2007–2008 SHM survey, residents or

Exhibit 4.2   Potential Residency Training Sources for Hospitalist Candidates

Residency training programs may serve as a source for your hospitalist program. These training programs may be:

- Primary care based (with or without a hospitalist track)
  ○ Internal medicine or internal medicine–pediatrics
  ○ Family medicine
  ○ Pediatric
- Subspecialty based
  ○ Intensivists
  ○ Pulmonologists
  ○ Cardiologists
- Hospitalist fellowship
- Emergency medicine–based

---

fellows represent 50% of the candidate pool, candidates from another hospitalist program represent 28%, and candidates from a different field of medicine (e.g., nonhospitalists) represent 19%.

There are many factors to consider when deciding which type of candidate to recruit. For example, do you want an experienced hospitalist, or do you want to recruit someone fresh out of residency? Do you want to recruit an established physician in the community who will have a great understanding of the needs of referring outpatient providers? Would you consider a subspecialist who is equipped with a vast amount of knowledge (and skills) in one field but may not have the primary care exposure to meet all the patients' needs? There are pros and cons for each choice and we will put some forward for your consideration.

Experienced Hospitalists

Established hospitalists are an excellent recruitment choice in most instances. They bring experience and may expose your program to new ways of doing things. These physicians are also accustomed to the pace of hospitalist medicine (e.g., "seasoned veterans"). Additionally, there should be less training involved during the orientation process and less overtime. Conversely, experienced hospitalists may have developed bad habits that your program will need to break. In addition, they may be in need of a job for nefarious reasons. For example, they may have been fired or forced to resign due to personality conflicts, incompetency, lack of productivity, inappropriate or unprofessional behavior, or poor attendance.

During the interview process, explore why this person is looking at other programs. For example, are there any issues between the candidate and the current employer of which you should be aware? Does the candidate bring any "baggage"? Will your opportunity serve as a stepping-stone, or is it being used as leverage? Finally, if your program is financially strapped, you must consider the cost (salary and political) that your program will incur to recruit an experienced hospitalist. Some candidates may make more money than your salary scale allows. Bringing a new physician into the practice at a higher salary than those of some of your currently employed physicians may cause resentment among physicians and animosity toward the administrative team as a whole.

New Residency Graduates

There are some special factors to consider when you interview a graduate just finishing residency. The advantages of hiring a new grad include the fact that they are usually more malleable than experienced physicians, who may be set in their ways. New graduates are typically energetic, openminded, and welcome guidance. These candidates bring both a wealth of current knowledge and exposure to the latest technologies. Finally, new graduates may cost your program less money in salary, although this may be neutralized if they have a significant amount of medical school loans.

On the negative side, new graduates usually require close supervision and guidance, which may stretch your program's resources. The mindset of a recent graduate may take time to acclimate to that of an attending physician. This adjustment must also include education regarding both the financial and practice management aspects of medicine (e.g., coding, documentation, appropriate resource utilization). They must also become skilled at customer service as it relates both to the patient and to a referring provider.

Established Physicians in Community Practices

Recruitment of established physicians in private practice can be an excellent choice for your program. Established physicians typically have an understanding of the financial and practice management aspects of medicine (although some doctors may be leaving because they are failing in these aspects of their practice). Additionally, they are sensitive to demands placed on the outpatient physician. These physicians also appreciate the long-term relationship that has developed between the PCP and the patient. As a result, they can offer a referring provider–hospitalist partnership predicated on communication, continuity of care, and mutual respect. This is very helpful from a customer satisfaction perspective. Finally, community physicians are aware of services available to patients upon discharge, which can have a positive impact on clinical outcomes.

When interviewing nonhospitalist candidates, query their decision to leave private practice. Are they using this opportunity to slow down professionally and ride off into the sunset? Do they actively practice inpatient medicine? If so, what is their average inpatient census? Can they keep up with the pace, and are they ready to buy into the hospitalist model of inpatient care? Some physicians who transition into the hospital do not change their approach to the patient. For example, they may arrive at work midmorning, make hospital rounds once each day, and leave the hospital after all patients have been examined. The hospitalist model typically calls for arrival in the early morning, rounds twice a day, with availability late in the afternoon for conferences with the nursing staff and/or families.

As noted earlier, exhibit caution when recruiting an established physician from within the community, as there may be potential political ramifications for your program. For example, physicians in a local practice may be offended if you recruit a physician from their practice. In addition, if the candidate has a poor reputation in the community or hospital, it could hurt referrals into your program and/or have a negative impact on the hospital's support for your practice. On the other hand, if the candidate has an excellent reputation, it could inspire confidence in the hospitalist program and lead to an increase in referrals.

Primary Care–Based Physicians vs. Subspecialists

Adult hospitalist programs must decide which specialties make excellent hospitalists. Although there are many fine choices, most would agree that primary care–based physicians have the necessary communication skills and training to flourish in the role of hospitalist. As discussed in Chapter 2, the majority of hospitalists currently are physicians trained in general internal medicine. As the demand for hospitalists increases and the pool of internists decreases, physicians trained in both family medicine and internal medicine–pediatric will be in greater demand. The pros and cons of each of these specialties were discussed in Chapter 2. It is worth noting that choice of a given specialty may depend on the culture of your medical community and hospital.

Some hospitalist programs recruit subspecialists as part of their team. There are advantages to having intensivists or pulmonologists in your practice, especially if the hospital has a closed intensive care unit (ICU) that allows only subspecialists to practice in this unit. It is also advantageous if your program has a large number of critically ill patients and/or if the hospital is a tertiary care center that receives numerous transfers from the outlying areas (that are admitted to your program).

Emergency Department Physicians

Emergency medicine–trained physicians may make good hospitalists. These doctors, by the nature of their training, are very comfortable treating critically ill patients. Many of them also possess excellent procedural skills, such as placing central lines and intubating patients. Some ED physicians are internal medicine or family medicine trained, making them excellent hospitalist candidates. These providers possess knowledge and sensitivity of the demands and needs of the ED physician as well as those of the hospitalist if they have worked in a hospital utilizing such a program. The major drawback is that many emergency medicine–trained physicians do not have experience *managing* the care of patients.

Locum Tenens Physicians

Some hospitalist locum tenens physicians accept an assignment with the intention of evaluating the professional opportunity and community for permanent employment. This phenomenon is becoming more common, a good example being the Society of Hospital Medicine town meeting held in Dallas in May 2007. This can have a win–win outcome, as it gives your program a chance to observe and evaluate a physician before making a decision.

International Medical Graduates

IMGs account for one-fourth of the nation's practicing physicians. Accordingly, IMG recruitment is becoming an increasingly popular choice across the country. As discussed in Chapter 1, many of these physicians find rural and suburban areas attractive due to their visa restrictions (e.g., J-1 visa status). Consequently, hospitalist programs in these geographic regions may have an advantage in recruiting an IMG candidate. Ultimately, a person's IMG training and visa status will influence your choice.

5 Challenges Recruiting Hospitalists

Despite the dramatic increase in the number of practicing hospitalists, successful recruitment and retention of these physicians remains a difficult proposition. It can be stated that the hospitalist profession is a buyer's market. Several dynamics contribute to this demand as noted earlier. Generally speaking, hospitalist popularity has risen dramatically over the last several years, and consequently, hospitalist responsibilities have expanded. This has led to employment of a great number of hospitalist physicians to serve in a variety of roles. Despite this increase in supply, current demand remains unmet.

There are several factors to consider when inviting a candidate to visit your program and community (see Exhibit 5.1). These considerations and the recruitment challenges that accompany them are probably far greater then any that you've experienced in the past. This is a result of the stiff competition in the hospitalist recruitment marketplace. The following are practice-related factors that any hospitalist program must consider prior to bringing a candidate to town.

5.1 PHYSICIAN COMPENSATION

A competitive compensation package will allow your hospitalist program to attract exceptional candidates. There are many factors to consider when designing a physician compensation package. These include budgetary limitations, geographic considerations (e.g., what the local competition is paying, whether your location warrants paying a premium in salary to attract candidates), financial considerations (e.g., the amount of hospital subsidy your program receives), physician productivity and revenue generated (e.g., physician workload projections), as well as program deliverables offered (e.g., the scope of physician responsibilities). The information that follows was taken from the

Hospitalist Recruitment and Retention: Building a Hospital Medicine Program,
By Kenneth G. Simone
Copyright © 2010 Wiley-Blackwell

Exhibit 5.1 Practice-Related Factors Affecting Recruitment and Retention

Candidates will assess several aspects (clinical and nonclinical) of your practice opportunity before reaching a decision. The relative importance of these aspects will vary for each physician. Following are some practice-related factors that will affect a candidate's choice of employment:

- Salary and benefits
- Practice model
- Work hours/call schedule
- Daily workload
- Expectations/demands from the hospital
- Medical staff support
  ○ Specialty providers
  ○ Referral network
- Hospital administrative support
- Hospital staff culture and support
- Hospital systems
- Program staffing/program stability
- Empowerment and career path
- Community and practice culture

Society of Hospital Medicine survey in 2007–2008 (using the unadjusted data) and provides a starting point to establish fair market value (with comparisons to the 2005–2006 survey shown in parentheses).

Mean total compensation
    Adult: $188.5 K ($171.1 K)
    Pediatric: $154.5 K ($146 K)
    Adult–pediatric: $184.7 K ($188.5 K)

Whereas mean compensation increased in the latest survey (excluding adult–pediatric physicians), mean encounters per year and mean collections decreased compared to the 2005–2006 survey. This may imply that hospitalists are getting paid more to do less work since the last SHM survey. In reality, it may indicate that hospitalists are providing more nonbillable services (thus the increase in pay), which cannot be measured by encounters or billable events. For example, a hospitalist program may hire an additional physician to assist with additional services that the practice has assumed (e.g., in-house night call). Although the number of hospitalist patients may not increase (e.g., the same number of admissions per night as before), the number of physicians has increased to provide the services, and thus the number of encounters or patient charges has actually decreased per provider.

Mean adult total compensation by employment model
    Hospital employed: $189.7 K ($173 K)
    Academic: $168.8 K ($157 K)
    Management company: $215 K ($161 K)
    Local private hospitalist groups: $211.1 K ($172 K)
    Multispecialty groups: $196.7 K ($179 K)

In the latest survey, hospitalists in private practice groups worked more hours, were more productive, and earned more in total compensation (including benefits) than other models. It may be postulated that by the nature of their employment model, private hospitalists have an incentive to work harder. Conversely, academic hospitalists worked fewer hours, were less productive, and made less in total compensation. This is consistent with the fact that academic hospitalists divide their time between teaching–clinical activities and research, thus limiting their patient contact and productivity. When analyzing total encounters per year, hospitalists employed by management companies were most productive, followed by hospitalists in private practice.

Mean pediatric total compensation by employment model
    Hospital employed: $165.7 K
    Academic: $149.9 K

Hospital-employed pediatric hospitalists were less productive (e.g., RVUs), had fewer encounters per year, yet made more than academic hospitalists while working the same number of hours. There were only four survey responses for three categories of employment models, and thus the implication of these data is unknown.

Mean adult compensation by geographic region
    East: $181.9 K ($166 K)
    South: $196.3 K ($182 K)
    Midwest: $194.7 K ($161 K)
    West: $184 K ($160 K)

Analysis of compensation by region indicated that hospitalists in the South and Midwest had more encounters (mean) per year and received greater compensation than did physicians in the East and West. It would be logical to conclude that the higher productivity in the South and Midwest was responsible for the greater compensation enjoyed in these geographic regions.

Mean pediatric compensation by geographic region
    East: $148 K
    South: $158.4 K
    Midwest: $165.6 K
    West: $128.5 K

Pediatric hospitalists in the Midwest had the most encounters per year and received the highest compensation, and those in the West had the second-most encounters per year, billed the least amount, and received the lowest compensation among the four regions.

Type of compensation arrangement (adult and pediatrics)
    Salary only: 25% (27%)
    Productivity/performance based: 4% (4%)
    Mixed salary and productivity/performance based: 70% (68%)

Analysis of compensation arrangements indicate that 57% of pediatric programs and 46% of academic programs had their physicians on straight salary, while 91% of management company physicians were on a mixed salary- and productivity/performance–based arrangement. These compensation arrangements make sense because the number of annual encounters (and productivity) for pediatric programs tend to be lower than for adult programs. Thus, incentive-based productivity would be difficult for pediatric hospitalists to realize unless the targets were lowered considerably. It may follow that there would be less money available to reward these pediatricians.

It is more difficult to evaluate academicians' productivity when a good portion of their time is dedicated to teaching and research. As with pediatricians, annual encounters are fewer and productivity is less compared to other hospitalist models. In comparison, hospitalists employed by management companies have the greatest number of annual encounters and RVUs, and the majority are partially compensated based on their productivity and performance. One may surmise that high productivity is a consequence of their compensation model (although this is not known for certain).

The data above were presented to provide the reader with a general idea of hospitalist marketplace compensation. Numerous compensation arrangements can be created and customized for your program. In general, a competitive salary with opportunity for a performance-based bonus (referred to in this book as an *incentive plan*) is attractive to most physicians and may make your employment opportunity more appealing. In a recent survey performed by Cejka, 32% of those leaving a practice did so to seek higher compensation [10]. Incentive plans are discussed in detail in Chapter 6.

5.2   PRACTICE MODEL

Practice structure is becoming increasingly important to hospitalist candidates. Models that avoid traditional 36-hour shifts (e.g., rotating night call) and/or offer several consecutive days off (e.g., seven-on/seven-off block schedule) are currently popular. Schedules that eliminate night call (e.g., shifts of 24 hours or more) are also attractive. This can be accomplished through the creation of a rotating night shift or by hiring nocturnists (physicians who work only at night). Next, we discuss several factors to consider prior to choosing a particular scheduling model.

Continuity of Care

Continuity of care and communication (among all members of the healthcare team) support successful clinical outcomes, patient satisfaction, and referring provider satisfaction. For example, if providers work in a shift-based schedule, there is increased risk for communication breakdown and loss of continuity of care. In this model, providers may be scheduled arbitrarily to work a day, evening, or night shift. The shifts often vary from day to day (e.g., without regard to consecutive shifts), which may fragment both the physician's schedule and patient care. A similar model is employed in the ED, where continuity of care is not an issue. The advantages of this schedule include schedule flexibility and the absence of night call. The major disadvantages are loss of teamwork, communication, and continuity of care.

Schedule Flexibility

Schedule flexibility is very important for today's hospitalist. As discussed in Chapter 1, new graduates (e.g., genX'ers and the millennial generation) value highly both family and personal time. They seek job opportunities offering work–life balance (e.g., quality of life), and thus are attracted to programs with flexible schedules (including job sharing and part-time positions) and minimal night call burden.

Block scheduling can offer a hospitalist program flexibility. There are many variations of this type of scheduling model. In a seven-on/seven-off model, hospitalists are divided into two-physician teams. One physician from each team is scheduled to work for seven consecutive days followed by seven days off. Each team member transfers his or her patients to the other member when the seven days are completed. The team rotation is staggered so that all providers do not change at one time. There is also a person assigned to night call. All physicians rotate onto the night call slot throughout the year unless the program hires a team of nocturnists.

This model appears to provide continuity of care, which will support successful clinical outcomes. It also offers the highly desirable lifestyle flexibility. Physicians work 26 weeks each year and have 26 weeks off. Many programs provide two weeks of vacation time, thus lowering the number of workweeks per year to 24. This schedule may appear less cost-effective than others because at any given time only half the providers are working. This model can actually save money for a hospitalist program because it supports recruitment and retention of hospitalists, which stabilizes the practice (e.g., decreases physician turnover). Remember, recruitment costs for a new physician can approximate well over $100,000 [11]. The disadvantage of this model is having only one-half of the hospitalists work at any given time, which will limit patient capacity (e.g., daily census) for the program and may have a negative impact on the added-value services that the hospitalists can provide.

A variation of block scheduling requires multiple physicians to work in the daytime, one provider to work at night, and some combination to work the weekend. Blocks are staggered so that more physicians work in the hospital at any one time than with the seven-on/seven-off schedule. This schedule allows for 8- to 14-hour shifts, resulting in no "call" requirements (e.g., no 24- or 26-hour shifts). Physicians are scheduled in blocks comprised of 4 to 14 consecutive days or nights followed by a number of days off. The schedule typically rotates so that each provider covers days, nights, and weekends throughout the year. The blocks usually rotate every two to six weeks. The advantages of this model include continuity of care, lack of call, and the increased availability of physicians within the hospital. This allows for increased patient capacity, translating into a larger ADC. This staggered block schedule may foster greater communication among stakeholders and result in more cost-effective medical care. The disadvantage occurs in the potential for provider burnout and turnover, depending on the length of the blocks.

In summary, practice models that are flexible, enhance quality of life, and avoid burnout will support successful recruitment and retention of hospitalist physicians. Part-time opportunities are on the rise and may further improve physician satisfaction. The proportion of physicians working part-time increased from 13% (15% men and 8% women) in 2005 to 19% in 2007 (7% men and 12% women) [12]. In their survey, Cejka reported that flexible work hours and/or part-time options were one of the top three ongoing retention initiatives by medical groups.

Efficiency

The efficiency of a particular practice model can vary depending on the number of providers in the practice. For example, if a four-physician program were to utilize a seven-on/seven-off model with one hospitalist working in the day and one working at night, the program would effectively be paying four physicians to cover an ADC suitable for one physician. This would limit the number of participating outpatient practices (referring patients to the hospitalist practice), the scope of services provided, and the ability for program growth. The subsidy required to run the practice would also be high.

If the program utilized a rotating call model where three providers worked each week and one provider was off, this would increase the capacity and efficiency of the program. It should also decrease the amount of subsidy required to run the program. The practice model and daily work schedule should be matched appropriately with the number of providers in the program.

Physician Staffing

The schedule model in many instances is guided by the number of physicians in the hospitalist program. For example, a seven-on/seven-off model would not work if the program has only three or four providers. In that case the program may need to use a rotating call schedule (e.g., the traditional model) where all members of the practice are required to cover night calls and weekends on a regular rotating basis. Thus, each provider will work a 24- or 36-hour shift on a rotating basis (considering the day-shift responsibilities the day of and after a call).

Some practices allow the hospitalist to go home early after making rounds the morning following a call. Weekends can either be shared (increasing the number of disrupted weekends for each provider) or covered by one physician. This model is cost-effective, maintains continuity of care, and fosters communication. Scheduling flexibility will vary depending on the number of hospitalist physicians in the practice. The down side of this model is that night calls and weekends can be overwhelmingly busy. Quality-of-life concerns are not addressed with traditional call. This is one of the least attractive models for hospitalists and may be a setup for burnout and, ultimately, increased practice turnover.

Scope of Hospitalist Services Offered

A hospitalist program's scope of service may affect both the number of physicians within a program and the scheduling model. Conversely, both the number of hospitalists and the program's scheduling model may affect the scope of services offered. If the sponsoring hospital solicits the program to provide added-value services, the hospital typically provides a subsidy for nonreimbursable services. This subsidy provides additional revenue for the program, which may be budgeted for additional staff to grow the program. If the sponsoring hospital does not provide a subsidy, the program may have a difficult decision regarding the scope of services offered. A lack of hospital subsidy may negatively affect both staffing numbers and scheduling model.

To illustrate this point, if the hospital requests 24/7 in-house coverage, the cost of the hospitalist program will increase because more providers are typically needed to provide continuous on-site coverage. Nighttime work creates not create the revenue that daytime work creates (e.g., routine patient rounding does not occur at night; thus there are fewer patient contacts). This adds to the overall financial burden on the program. A subsidy will be required from the hospital to provide this service. In addition to hiring additional providers, the program may need to adjust the scheduling model, as most 24/7 programs utilize a block schedule, to provide continuous coverage.

5.3   WORK AND CALL SCHEDULE

In addition to the practice model, candidates will be very interested to learn about the structure of the workday and the frequency of both night and weekend call. For example, they will be curious about the start of the workday, whether there are midday or late shifts (e.g., float shift), as well as the length of the workday (e.g., hours per day). The typical hospitalist shift runs anywhere from 8 to 14 hours in duration. Midday and swing or late shifts may be attractive to the hospitalist, as they will receive support during the busiest times of the workday. Candidates are also interested to know whether there is night call (e.g., as opposed to a night shift), as well as the frequency of weekend call. Programs employing nocturnists will have an overall advantage in recruitment. Keep in mind that 17% of the time a physician's departure from a practice is a result of an incompatible work schedule and excessive call schedule [10].

During the site visit, discuss how the program covers holidays, vacation time, and extended leave (e.g., maternity or paternity leave, sick leave). Candidates will want to hear details about coverage and how it will affect them. Inform the candidate if coverage is provided by moonlighters or from within the practice (e.g., internal moonlighting).

5.4   DAILY WORKLOAD

The daily workload is another point of interest for candidates. Everyone has heard the saying "If it sounds too good to be true, it probably is." Some programs offer hospitalist candidates a significant sign-on bonus, moving expenses, medical school loan repayment, a considerable salary, and significant time off each year. When the candidate digs deeper he or she will typically find that the daily workload is unmanageable. Some programs expect physicians to see 25 to 30 or more patients per day in addition to their nonclinical responsibilities. These providers may be required to meet national benchmarks for ALOS, utilization, and patient outcomes (e.g., readmission rates, morbidity and mortality rates). Many programs offset these large financial packages by cutting down on the number of hospitalists in the practice. Make no mistake; if the workload is unmanageable, the hospitalist will leave the program at the first opportunity.

Candidates will be interested in discussing daily workload as it relates to average daily census per provider, physician staffing per shift, the presence or absence of support staff (e.g., NPCs, dedicated case managers, nonclinical hospitalist staff), and the extent of nonclinical responsibilities. All of these factors should be discussed during the site visit.

5.5   ADDED-VALUE BENEFITS

Most hospitalist programs provide added-value benefits to their hospital. The specific deliverables vary from hospital to hospital and program
to program. The type and extent of these services can influence the
candidate's decision-making process. For example, does the program
provide call coverage for unassigned emergency department patients?
Do the hospitalists offer surgical co-management services? Do they
provide rapid-response team and/or code blue coverage? Do they
cover an observation unit or provide long-term acute care services?
Additionally and perhaps more important, how do hospital administration, the medical staff, hospital staff, and hospital systems support the
successful implementation of these services by the hospitalist program?
In Section 11.6 we explore collaborative systems in detail.

5.6   MEDICAL STAFF SUPPORT

The culture of the medical staff also influences hospitalist recruitment
and retention. A medical staff that works collegially and supports the
hospitalist program will have an advantage over those that are unsup-
portive. Supportive physicians in this instance may be defined as those
who refer patients to the hospitalist program and are readily available
to the hospitalists (e.g., to provide consultation, to provide hospitalist
coverage during times of need). In some medical communities, referring provider support may be fragile at best. The hospitalists may be
treated like glorified house officers or residents by the medical staff.
This can lead to missed opportunities with candidates.

5.7   HOSPITAL CULTURE AND SYSTEMS

Hospitals that boast an integrated healthcare delivery system will
have a positive impact on recruitment and retention. In an integrated
network, the medical staff works collaboratively with all healthcare
professionals. In the case of hospitalists, this collaboration typically
includes the development of multidisciplinary programs involving the
hospitalist physicians and nursing, case management, social service,
and pharmacy departments. The hospitalist physician is at the hub of
this network and in a great position to lead the institution. This can
provide professional challenges and create career opportunities that
support job satisfaction.

Workplace stability should be reviewed with all candidates. For example, if the hospital has a reputation of retaining its best nurses, this should be mentioned. If the hospital has dedicated case managers for the hospitalist program, this should be presented. If the hospital has received awards (e.g., patient safety, quality of care), this should be shared as well. The hospital's mission, long-term vision, objectives, and values should also be reviewed.

5.8 TECHNOLOGY

The latest SHM survey indicates that 50% of new hospitalists come straight from residency or fellowship programs. These new graduates have considerable exposure to the latest diagnostic and therapeutic technologies. In many instances these newly trained physicians rely heavily on new technologies. They may feel out of their "comfort zone" if these resources are not available. New graduates also have extensive knowledge of biostatistics and exposure to electronic medical records (EMRs). Access to an excellent data tracking system and EMRs will aid physicians in their quest for clinical excellence and may represent a recruitment advantage for your program.

Data tracking systems will be important from another perspective. Hospitalists live in a world of data collection, metrics, and benchmarking. Data may be used to evaluate a physician's performance and to allocate performance-based funds. This evaluation is dependent on the program's accurate and timely collection and analysis of data. Physicians will need access to this data to gauge their performance and modify their behavior appropriately. Many metrics are used to assess clinical and financial performance, including but not limited to clinical outcomes (morbidity and mortality rates, readmission rates), productivity (e.g., RVUs), utilization (e.g., ALOS, average cost per case), and compliance (e.g., the Joint Commission Core Measures, CMS pay-for-performance measures, utilization of evidence-based guidelines). If your program and/or sponsoring hospital offers a sophisticated data tracking system (and process), this should be discussed with the candidate.

5.9 SPECIALTY PROVIDERS

Composition of the medical staff can be a deciding factor for many hospitalist candidates. Generally speaking, a medical community that offers a wide range of subspecialty services attracts more candidates. However, some hospitalists welcome the opportunity to assume greater responsibilities, particularly in rural communities. The type of subspecialties represented and number of physicians in each (e.g., accessibility) may be an important factor in recruitment. For example, if the hospitalists are expected to care for closed-head injuries because of the absence of neurosurgeons, or if they are expected to admit patients for the gastroenterologists three days per week (due to a shortage of these physicians), the practice opportunity may be less attractive. The existence of co-management programs (e.g., orthopedic) can also be a factor in a candidate's decision-making process. It is prudent to be upfront with all candidates regarding the composition of the existing medical staff, presenting both their strengths and their limitations from the onset.

5.10   REFERRAL NETWORK

Hospitalist candidates will be interested to learn about the established relationships between the hospitalist practice and referral network. The referral network may consist of NPCs and physicians (e.g., PCPs and specialists). These relationships are crucial to the stability of any hospitalist program. If an adversarial relationship exists, recruitment can be affected negatively. When a collegial relationship is present, recruitment and retention will be easier to achieve. In addition to discussing existing relationships, it will be worthwhile to review the referral network's level of commitment to the hospitalist program (e.g., the number of admissions by both practice group and provider). If your program enjoys strong referral support, this should be emphasized. This emphasis serves to highlight job security to the candidate. This is especially important if there are competing hospitalist programs in the same community, either at the same hospital or at different institutions. Referring physician participation in the recruitment process will underscore the close working relationship the program enjoys with these doctors.

Referring physician satisfaction data (in the form of surveys) should also be shared with the candidate. If satisfaction is high, these surveys will reinforce the quality of the hospitalist program. Customer satisfaction also indicates program stability and collegial support. When there are problems with customer satisfaction, it is valuable to share the program's perspective and discuss the performance improvement plan.

5.11 HOSPITAL ADMINISTRATIVE SUPPORT

Candidates will critically evaluate the sponsoring hospital's level of commitment to the program. Hospital support may come in the form of funding (e.g., program subsidy for various services provided by the hospitalists), staffing (e.g., dedicated case managers, dedicated nursing staff), and/or practice resources [e.g., dedicated office space, hospitalist call room, computers, personal digital assistants (PDAs) Blackberries, funding for front-office staff]. Support may also come in the form of a collaborative relationship between hospital administration and the hospitalist program. For example, in some institutions a hospital administrator will meet monthly with the hospitalist clinical director. Some hospitals reserve a seat on the medical executive committee for hospitalist representation. Hospitals may also provide an annual joint strategic planning process (e.g., in the form of a retreat) with the hospitalist program (see Chapter 2). If any of these initiatives exists at your institution, they should be discussed with the candidate in detail. Hospitalist programs that enjoy a close working relationship with hospital administration will be more attractive to candidates.

5.12 STAFF STABILITY

The stability of the hospitalist clinical staff is crucial to the overall performance of the practice. If a program is understaffed, it will destabilize the practice, making recruitment and retention more of a challenge. For example, when a program is understaffed, fewer physicians will be available to care for the same number of patients. This will make it difficult for these doctors to practice in a cost-effective manner while providing good-quality medical care. As a result, ALOS and resource utilization may rise, adding to the pressure that these physicians are already experiencing.

These adverse effects will be similar in unstable programs characterized by continual physician turnover. In this situation physician *continuity* is lost due to the changing roster of providers, which will disrupt both the culture and dynamics of the practice. This has a negative effect on the program's ability to standardize care, which may affect both the quality and efficiency of care rendered. It is worth noting that chronically understaffed programs tend to experience high physician turnover. Candidates tend to avoid understaffed and/or unstable programs.

If your program is experiencing staffing problems, take the time to discuss this openly with the candidate. For example, the problem may be that your program's in a growth mode, which is a perfectly acceptable reason to be understaffed. More important, communicate the strategic plan in place to address this challenge. Candidates may find an understaffed employment opportunity attractive if there are ample provisions for interim coverage and a long-term strategy for appropriate staffing.

5.13 COMMUNITY AND PRACTICE CULTURE

In the Cejka survey cited earlier, community fit, practice fit, and practice culture are the most common factors influencing physician retention. In this survey, 51% of people leaving a community did so because of poor cultural fit. It is thus critically important to clearly define the hospitalist program's mission, vision, and objectives, as well as to describe the hospital and community culture. Finding an appropriate fit is essential for program stability and physician job satisfaction.

Community fit is a very important factor for the candidate's spouse and family as well. Many physicians who leave their practice voluntarily do so secondary to family considerations. In many instances, spousal job relocation (22% in the Cejka survey) played a part in turnover. Proximity to family is also a factor. Thus, the focus of recruitment needs to include the spouse or significant other in addition to the candidate. There are many recruitment and retention strategies addressing community and practice fit. The details of these strategies are discussed and defined in Chapters 8 and 9.

In summary, there are various factors unique to your practice opportunity that will influence candidates in the recruitment process. The scheduling examples presented were a small sampling of how your practice model may be designed. There are many creative concepts that can be incorporated into the practice model or physician schedule to customize it. These concepts will support the delivery of quality care as well as the quality of life for your physicians. The initial practice model chosen may be just the beginning of an evolution in your practice model.

Finally, the success of your program will be influenced by the flexibility of the hospitalist practice management team, hospitalist providers, and physician schedule. Success is also predicated on building an integrated healthcare system that supports both the hospitalist program and its providers. The healthcare team (e.g., hospitalists, referring physicians, medical staff, hospital staff, hospital administration) should work collaboratively and share a similar vision of patient care. In the final analysis, the healthcare system must support the delivery of cost-effective, efficient, high-quality care while maintaining continuity of care and communication with all of its stakeholders.

6 Incentive Plans

Incentive programs are an extremely valuable tool to enhance recruitment and retention. These are designed to motivate (in the form of a reward) both individual and team (e.g., practice) performance. The metrics chosen typically support the program's strategic plan and objectives. In some instances a metric may be chosen to effect a change in behavior and/or gain buy-in for an initiative that may otherwise be met with resistance. Incentive programs also provide physicians with an opportunity to increase their earnings. When individual hospitalists achieve incentive objectives, the overall program will benefit.

There are many variations in incentive plan format and administration. Some programs offer group incentives, whereas others offer incentives based on individual performance. Mixed incentive programs (group and individual based) promote teamwork while rewarding individual performance. Some programs place a portion of the physician's salary at risk within the incentive plan (effectively creating a risk corridor).

There are several variables to consider during incentive plan creation. All of these variables can have an impact on the success or failure of the plan. Therefore, exhibit caution as you design the plan and be aware of the potential pitfalls. We address the key variables in Sections 6.1 through 6.5.

6.1   INCENTIVE PLAN OBJECTIVES

Incentive plan objectives are dynamic and should be evaluated on an annual basis. The objectives must be both clearly defined and attainable. The incentive objectives may address clinical and/or financial performance. They may address cultural or behavioral issues within the practice (e.g., customer service, operational, structural). They may also

Hospitalist Recruitment and Retention: Building a Hospital Medicine Program,
By Kenneth G. Simone
Copyright © 2010 Wiley-Blackwell

focus on a new service line initiative (e.g., palliative care program, observation bed management, surgery co-management program). Finally, the objectives may address regulatory initiatives. Some objectives warrant adjustments (at the end of the fiscal year) once they are realized. For example, if your providers were incentivized to *create* a palliative care program this past year and this was accomplished, you may create a new objective regarding *growth* or *performance* of the palliative care team for the coming year. Whatever the objective, keep it simple and make sure that it can be measured.

6.2   DATA SYSTEMS

Hospitalist programs must consider the limitations of the data tracking system before choosing specific incentive plan metrics. Effective data systems produce information that is accurate, accessible, reproducible, and timely. Common sources of data are the hospitalist program's billing data, and the hospital's clinical and financial information systems. Unfortunately, it is difficult for many hospitals (and hospitalist programs) to capture all of the information requested and to integrate it in a timely manner. Engage the hospital's information technology personnel from the onset to assist in this endeavor (see Information Technology Programs in Section 11.6).

Initiate targets that you know can easily be measured. If a metric cannot be measured directly but is felt to be essential to monitor performance (physician or team), it may be acceptable to use a proxy. Use a proxy only if all involved parties agree on the surrogate measure. If your physicians develop mistrust of the data, it can cause unraveling of the incentive plan, resulting in lower practice morale and negative physician performance.

6.3   METRICS

There are a number of metrics for consideration when building an incentive plan. Creating a plan that monitors a broad spectrum of performance (e.g., clinical, financial, operational) is prudent (see Exhibit 6.1). It is wise to avoid metrics that are difficult to measure or track. The incentive metrics should have significance in the form of impact for both the hospitalist program and the sponsoring hospital. In general, the metrics should monitor areas in need of improvement and areas critical to the success of the program. The information obtained from

Exhibit 6.1   Incentive Plan Metrics

Successful incentive plans typically choose a variety of metrics to assess both physician and practice performance. The selection of these metrics will vary according to a number of variables specific for each practice. These metrics allow your program to focus on problem areas within the practice. They also allow your program to place emphasis on areas vital to the program's success. These plans:

- Reward high-quality patient care and the practice of evidence-based medicine
- Emphasize continuity of care
- Emphasize communication with the patient and family, PCP, specialists, and healthcare team (e.g., nursing, case management, UR)
- Reward leadership
- Reward participation in practice management activities
- Reward appropriate coding and documentation
- Reward participation in added-value activities
- Stress teamwork and good citizenship
- Reward productivity
- Emphasize fiscal responsibility
- Emphasize customer satisfaction

The specific metrics chosen may assess a variety of performance areas: These areas can be divided into six categories. There are several potential measures worth consideration within each category. The choice of measure will depend on the performance of past practices as well as the future direction of the program. It will also be influenced by both the ease (e.g., accessibility of the data, timeliness of the process) and accuracy of measurement. The categories are as follows:

- *Clinical performance.* These indicators are typically based on two subgroups: clinical outcomes and the adherence to state and/or national initiatives from accreditation or regulatory agencies (e.g., the Joint Commission, CMS, the state). Indicators within this category are a very popular choice for incentive plans because they involve quality of care, regulatory compliance, and ultimately affect the bottom line. The clinical performance of the program may be measured by:

- Morbidity and mortality rate
- Readmission rate (72-hour and 30-day)
- Rate of unexpected return to the ICU
- Utilization of evidence-based clinical guidelines
- Compliance with Medicare–Joint Commission core measures (e.g., heart failure, pneumonia, acute myocardial infarction)
- Compliance with pay-for-performance measures
- Medication reconciliation
- Patient safety initiatives
- Compliance with the Joint Commission mandate regarding unacceptable abbreviations

- *Operational efficiency.* Some of the indicators in this category address interdisciplinary processes and performance. In many instances these indicators may be as much a measure of the existing (sponsoring) hospital systems as they are about the hospitalist program and providers. Examples of operational indicators include:
  - Compliance with hands-off protocols
  - Responsiveness to the nursing staff and ED (e.g., throughput issues)
  - Appropriate coding and chart documentation
- *Administrative responsibilities.* Indicators in this category focus on each hospitalist's performance concerning nonclinical responsibilities. Although this category does not directly involve clinical performance, it has a significant impact on the hospitalist program (e.g., financially), the hospitalists (e.g., their standing within the medical staff), and the hospital (e.g., Medicare billing requirements).
  - Timely dictation of the H/P and D/C summary
  - Timely completion of medical records
  - Timely submission of charges
  - Attendance at required meetings
- *Productivity.* This category directly addresses the work that physicians perform within the practice. The productivity indicators have a bearing on the bottom line of the program and are thus an area of great interest. Although many incentive plans place great emphasis on this category, the hospitalists are in part dependent on other sources (e.g., referring physicians) to generate work. The hospitalist's productivity will also be affected by

the shift worked (e.g., day, evening, night) and the role the hospitalist plays (e.g., admitter, rounder, nocturnist). Physician coding (although an operational indicator) will affect productivity as well.

○ RVUs
○ Annual billable encounters

- *Customer service.* As with all businesses, customer service and satisfaction are both very important indicators of employee performance. As hospitalists, these physicians serve many customers. Satisfaction among all stakeholders is essential to the overall success of the program. If the physicians fall short in this category, it may cause instability within the program and sponsoring hospital. This may doom the hospitalist program to failure. A number of factors are included:

○ Patient satisfaction
○ Referring provider satisfaction
○ Nursing department and ED satisfaction
○ Establishing collaborative relationships with key stakeholders
○ Acceptance of admissions and transfers

- *Leadership, teamwork, and good citizenship.* In many ways this category is what separates hospitalist physicians from other doctors on the medical staff in hospitals. This category is often referred to as the *added-value services* that hospitalists provide to the medical community and sponsoring institution. These services are invaluable to the hospital, hospital staff, and medical staff. Although it is difficult to place a monetary value on them, it is advantageous to reward the hospitalists' work as it relates to these services.

○ Adherence to practice policies, procedures, and protocols
○ Participation on the code blue and rapid-response teams
○ Participation in multidisciplinary morning rounds
○ Serving in a medical staff leadership role
○ Serving on key medical staff committees
○ Creating evidence-based clinical guidelines and order sets
○ Teaching residents and medical students
○ Participation in educational initiatives with the hospital staff (e.g., nursing department, ED)

this process should be tangible, providing feedback that can be utilized for performance improvement by both the hospitalist program and the hospital. In addition to providing performance feedback, incentive plans can guide the future direction of the hospitalist program.

It is useful to review national initiatives prior to instituting clinical performance-based measures. Frequently, quality organizations such as the National Quality Forum, IHI, and Leapfrog create new and innovative clinical initiatives that may benefit both the hospitalist program and the sponsoring hospital. In addition, regulatory agencies frequently create new initiatives (e.g., CMS pay-for-performance, "never event" initiatives) that can be incorporated.

When creating your incentive program, consider selecting one to two metrics from each of the six categories outlined in Exhibit 6.1. Each category must then be weighted according to program importance (the focus and specific metrics may change annually). For example, your program may decide to focus on improving clinical quality and customer service the first year. The metrics may be weighted as follows: clinical, 40%; customer service, 25%; productivity, 15%; operational, 10%; administrative, 5%; and leadership 5%. Thus each quarter, physicians will have an opportunity to receive one-fourth of the bonus in each category. Each metric can either be administered in an "all or none" manner (e.g., must hit the designated target), which is highly recommended, or it may be tiered. In a tiered approach, if the physician reaches 50% of the benchmark (e.g., the benchmark for medical record completion may be 80% within two weeks of discharge and the provider performs at a 40% rate), one-half of the potential monies for that metric in that quarter will be distributed. If the physician reaches 75% of the benchmark, three-fourths of the monies will be distributed, and so on.

If your program has selected productivity (e.g., RVUs) as an incentive metric, accommodations must be made regarding the targets for nocturnists. These physicians will be less productive by the nature of their job. Your program can use historical data to establish a benchmark for these doctors from data previously available (preferred route). For example, if past data suggest that your nighttime physicians are only 65% as productive as the daytime hospitalists, you can lower the RVU target to 65% of the other doctors. If data are not available (e.g., a new program), you may decide to raise the nocturnist's base salary and keep the targets the same for all hospitalists. You may also use national benchmarks (e.g., from the SHM survey) to guide this metric. Part-time hospitalists should also have their productivity targets modified according to the number of hours they work (e.g., the RVU target for a one-half FTE should be 50% that of a full-time hospitalist).

It is worth mentioning that hospitalist programs should use caution when deciding which metrics to include in the incentive plan. Plans that are based on number of admissions, daily census, and gross/net charges, for example, may provide an incentive for the physician to admit more patients and keep them in the hospital longer. Plans that rewards reduced length of stay (or reduced average cost per case) may provide an incentive for the physician to discharge patients prematurely, resulting in suboptimal clinical outcomes and an increased risk of readmission. This runs counterintuitive to what hospitalist programs are trying to accomplish. Development of a robust case management program may safeguard against these concerns.

6.4   BENCHMARKING

Performance targets (e.g., best practice benchmarks) must be established once metrics have been chosen. These targets can be created after reviewing historical data of peer group performance in similar categories. The peer group may be local or the data may be obtained from national organizations such as SHM and MGMA, or from independent repositories such as Solucient and Premier. Whatever the source, the targets must be reasonable. Setting unreachable goals will be counterproductive to what the practice is trying to accomplish. Making the goals too easy to reach will undermine the purpose of the incentive plan. SHM's white paper entitled "Measuring Hospitalist Performance: Metrics, Reports, and Dashboards" [32] is an excellent reference for programs building incentive programs and/or performance scorecards.

6.5   INCENTIVE PAYOUT

It is beneficial to understand the motivation of your hospitalist physicians when creating the incentive reward. For the most part, monetary incentives are a great motivator (although they may not be the sole motivator). Other performance and behavioral motivators include additional paid time off from work, schedule flexibility, workplace amenities (e.g., Blackberry, PDA, laptop, dedicated office workspace, dedicated call room), acknowledgment, and praise. If your financial resources are limited, these other incentives may be (more) attractive to your physicians.

As stated previously, incentive monies are typically paid out on a quarterly basis. This schedule provides the physician with regular feedback and facilitates performance improvement throughout the year. The amount of this incentive should be large enough to affect both physician behavior and performance. Some sources recommend an incentive amount of at least 10% of the base salary per year to effect meaningful change in performance.

Most programs provide equal distribution (e.g., payout percentage) for each metric pertaining to all the hospitalist physicians within the practice. However, keep in mind that every physician possesses his or her individual strengths and weaknesses. Furthermore, the purpose of the incentive plan is to ensure both the best quality and optimal financial outcome for the patient and program. Thus, your program may consider weighing each metric differently according to the past performance of each physician. For example, if a provider's performance is substandard for one metric, consider weighing a greater percentage of the incentive payout toward that metric. This will allow your program to customize the incentive disbursement for each metric in order to maximize the performance of each person and effect change. This manner of weighted distribution may also cause a logistical problem for the incentive plan administrator. The incentive program may be structured in many ways, depending on the culture of the practice. Following are examples of the more common incentive plan structures.

Traditional Incentive Plan

In a traditional plan, hospitalists receive a bonus based on individual performance (e.g., independent of practice associates). Thus, a person's substandard performance does not affect fellow hospitalists. The advantage of this plan is such that motivated and high-performing physicians will not be penalized for the substandard performance provided by the other hospitalists. The disadvantage of this type of incentive plan is that it does not reward the performance of the team as a whole (e.g., does not support teamwork).

Tiered Incentive Plan

In a tiered plan, the first tier defines team performance targets that must be attained by all physicians prior to recognition of individual achievement. Thus, if one physician falls short of the team targets, none is eligible for incentive monies during the quarter. Team targets are typically easily achievable but essential to the success of the practice. Examples of team targets include timely charge submission, timely medical record completion, and attendance at morning rounds. If all hospitalists reach the team targets, each physician is eligible for individual bonus money. The bonus is based on achieving additional individual performance targets (as with the traditional incentive plan). This plan creates peer pressure for all physicians in order to achieve basic performance standards. The advantage of this plan is that it supports both teamwork (at least for some metrics) and achievement of basic but necessary practice goals. The disadvantage is that the high-performing physicians may be penalized if any one physician's performance is substandard. This may eventually lead to physician malcontent and ultimately to turnover within the practice.

At-risk Plan

In an at-risk plan, a portion of the physician's salary is withheld at the beginning of the contract year. The money is placed into a pool with additional bonus dollars, thus creating a risk corridor. The physician may receive a quarterly bonus based on meeting the established performance benchmarks. The bonus may be "all-or none" each quarter or may be apportioned based on excellence. For example, if the physician reaches the 50th percentile in performance (as defined at the beginning of the year), 25% of the available bonus will be awarded; if the physician reaches the 75th percentile, 50% of the available bonus will be awarded; and if the physician reaches the 100th percentile, he or she will receive 100% of the quarterly bonus. The advantage of this plan is that it places a portion of the physician's baseline salary at risk. This may serve as a motivational factor similar to that of physicians in private practice (although a physician in private practice is totally at risk). The disadvantage is that it may deter some physicians from joining your practice, due to the uncertainty of a baseline salary. For many physicians, the security of a guaranteed salary is worth the loss of practice autonomy.

Team Bonus Pool

In a term pool plan, bonus money for the entire practice is placed in a pool and distributed quarterly to each physician based on individual performance. The money is allocated proportional to performance; thus, more deserving physicians receive a greater bonus. The advantage of this plan is that it creates competition among the hospitalist physicians, which may motivate individual performance. This is particularly true if your practice culture is such that the physicians are motivated by monetary reward. The disadvantage of this plan is that it may undermine teamwork. Specifically, it may do so by causing animosity and distrust among the hospitalist physicians. Use such a plan with caution and monitor the team chemistry closely.

In summary, effective incentive plans are well balanced and reward clinical performance. Clinical performance may be assessed, for example, by monitoring both patient morbidity and mortality rates and the rate of unexpected readmissions. It may also be assessed by monitoring adherence to evidence-based clinical guidelines, quality initiatives, and the Joint Commission's core measures.

Effective incentive plans also monitor and reward productivity (e.g., RVU-based), leadership, good citizenship (e.g., establish collaborative relationships with key stakeholders, exhibit professional behavior), and customer satisfaction (e.g., patient and referring physician). The metrics chosen should be easily measurable and the plan simple to implement. Selection of performance metrics is a dynamic process and should be reevaluated annually. Best practice benchmarks must be created to guide the physician's performance.

7 National Recruitment Initiatives

In the highly competitive marketplace of hospitalist recruitment, the benefits offered to hospitalist candidates may play a crucial role in winning over a candidate. The more creative your program can be regarding its benefit package offer, the greater chance you have to be successful in recruiting the candidate of your choice. For example, your program may have $20,000 at its disposal for recruitment enticements. If a candidate is established (e.g., has no medical school loans) and is located within a neighboring community, your program may offer the candidate all of this money in the form of a signing bonus. If the candidate is a new graduate, loan repayment may be more attractive than moving expenses. It is important to learn what each candidate values and attempt to match the benefits accordingly. Although flexibility is important, your program must use caution so that it does not set a precedent it cannot adhere to with other physicians in the program.

Over the last several years, Merritt, Hawkins and Associates (MHA), a major national recruitment firm, has performed an annual review exploring recruitment initiatives for *all specialties* and employment opportunities (13). The intent of the annual review is both to quantify financial and other incentives offered by employers and to identify those medical specialties in greatest demand. The data can also be used as a benchmark for those practices active in the recruitment marketplace. Samples of the findings are provided throughout the chapter.

Hospitalist Recruitment and Retention: Building a Hospital Medicine Program,
By Kenneth G. Simone
Copyright © 2010 Wiley-Blackwell

7.1   TREND IN HOSPITALIST SALARY (DOES NOT INCLUDE BONUS OR BENEFITS)

	Low	Average	High
2007–2008	$150,000	$181,000	$300,000
2006–2007	$145,000	$180,000	$250,000
2005–2006	$140,000	$175,000	$190,000
2004–2005	$150,000	$171,000	$210,000
2003–2004	$140,000	$162,000	$200,000

MHA's data on hospitalist salaries mirror SHM's findings that hospitalist salaries continue to trend upward, although the average salary in 2007–2008 is lower than what is reported in the SHM survey. It should be noted that it is not known how MHA defines a hospitalist, so direct comparisons cannot be made between these data. To illustrate this point, 2008 MGMA data indicated that the mean internal medicine hospitalist income was $201,830, but many doctors in this survey spent a portion of their time in an office-based setting. Thus, these data cannot be compared directly to SHM data.

Information concerning hospitalist salary should always be fully analyzed and put into perspective. For example, some programs offer a high salary without benefits; others may offer a moderate salary with an opportunity to earn significantly more money through an incentive plan, whereas others may offer a low base salary that is enhanced by an outstanding benefit plan. Additionally, income must be placed in perspective by considering the responsibilities of the hospitalists and how much work they perform.

7.2   TYPE OF INCENTIVES OFFERED FOR ALL SPECIALTIES

	Salary	Salary with Bonus	Income Guarantee
2007–2008	22%	59%	19%
2006–2007	12%	67%	21%
2005–2006	15%	53%	32%
2004–2005	10%	55%	35%
2003–2004	9%	50%	41%

MHA data indicate that a salary with a bonus is the most popular means of physician compensation, although the number of doctors paid by a straight salary increased significantly in 2007–2008. Keep in mind that these numbers reflect all specialties, and thus direct comparisons cannot be made to SHM's data. These data are included to illustrate physician compensation trends in general terms.

In 2008 (from May 7 to July 7), *Today's Hospitalist* performed a hospitalist compensation and career survey that further supported this trend in compensation. This survey indicated that with the exception of "university/medical school" hospitalist programs, all other hospitalist employment models (e.g., national management company, local hospitalist group, multispecialty primary care group, hospital-employed group) favored the combination salary and bonus/incentive compensation plan [14]. For example, approximately 68% of hospitalist management programs, 54% of local groups, 60% of multispecialty groups, and 68% of hospital-employed programs utilized the mixed compensation plan. University/medical school programs favored 100% salary compensation (e.g., 56% of programs).

Bonus plans vary considerably from program to program. Some are totally productivity based, whereas others reward various measures of performance, such as good citizenship, quality of care, and adherence to evidence-based clinical guidelines.

7.3   RELOCATION PAY, AND AMOUNT, FOR ALL SPECIALTIES

	Yes	No	Low	Average	High
2007–2008	92%	8%	$1,500	$9,807	$20,000
2006–2007	98%	2%	$1,000	$9,808	$75,000
2005–2006	99%	1%	$3,000	$10,060	$20,000
2004–2005	99%	1%	$3,500	$8,850	$20,000
2003–2004	99%	1%	$2,000	$9,250	$22,000

Most employment opportunities offer relocation (e.g., moving expense) reimbursement in the standard amount of $10,000. Relocation pay is quite common in the hospitalist marketplace; thus, it makes great sense for your program to offer this perk as a means of remaining competitive. Some programs require the physician to pay the expense upfront and provide reimbursement up to a predetermined amount of money (e.g., $10,000). In this way, if the moving expense is less than the allotted amount, the program would save money.

7.4 SIGNING BONUS, AND AMOUNT, FOR ALL SPECIALTIES

	Yes	No	Low	Average	High
2007–2008	74%	26%	$4,000	$24,800	$200,000
2006–2007	72%	28%	$5,000	$20,000	$100,000
2005–2006	58%	42%	$5,000	$20,480	$75,000
2004–2005	46%	54%	$5,000	$14,030	$50,000
2003–2004	50%	50%	$5,000	$15,500	$45,000

A sign-on bonus is another popular benefit offered to attract potential candidates. The average bonus in this review has increased annually over the past five years with the exception of 2006–2007. The average bonus listed by MHA in 2007–2008 appears high for hospitalist candidates, but the practice of offering one is strongly recommended. Some programs will pay one-half of the bonus at the time of the contract signing, one-fourth at midyear, and one-fourth at the end of the first year if the physician remains with the practice. In this way, the program retains a safety net in case the doctor leaves the practice prematurely.

7.5 AMOUNT OF CME FOR ALL SPECIALTIES

	Low	Average	High
2007–2008	$700	$3,924	$35,000
2006–2007	$1,000	$3,312	$15,000
2005–2006	$1,500	$3,830	$10,000
2004–2005	$1,000	$3,350	$15,000
2003–2004	$1,500	$3,250	$10,000

CME allowance is a common benefit provided by most hospitalist programs. In many programs the amount is granted according to years in the practice, with a typical ceiling of $5000. For example, physicians may receive $2500 in year one, $3000 in year two, $3500 in year three, $4000 in year four, and $5000 in year five and thereafter. Some programs provide additional monies for professional expenses such as medical license and medical journal subscriptions. Others may provide a cell phone, Blackberry, laptop, or PDA as an additional benefit to enhance communication within the practice.

7.6   ADDITIONAL BENEFITS

	2007–2008	2006–2007	2005–2006	2004–2005
Health insurance	95%	91%	91%	92%
Malpractice	96%	91%	92%	93%
Retirement	91%	72%	70%	72%
Disability	79%	69%	70%	74%
Educational loan forgiveness	35%	26%	34%	14%

With the tight economy in recent years, many physicians are looking for benefit packages that provide health and disability insurance, medical malpractice insurance, and a retirement plan (with profit share if applicable). If your program provides liability insurance, you should address upfront if a tail is provided with the malpractice policy. Some programs require the physician to pay 100% of the tail if they leave after the first year and decrease the amount to be paid by the physician over several years (see Chapter 10).

Other benefits may include life insurance and an option to become a partner or shareholder (e.g., if the employer is a private practice or management company). If the physician is a new graduate, medical school loan repayment is an excellent perk to attract candidates to your program. For example, some programs provide a fixed amount each year for three to five years. The program may provide a loan forgiveness policy that stipulates that monies do not need to be repaid if the physician stays an additional year with the practice for every year of loan repayment. For example, if the candidate receives three years of loan repayment and leaves the practice after working five years, he or she would be required to reimburse the third year of loan repayment.

7.7   HOSPITAL-EMPLOYED JOB OPPORTUNITIES

2007–2008	2006–2007	2005–2006	2004–2005
45%	43%	23%	19%

The number of hospital-employed physician job opportunities (per MHA data searches and the latest SHM survey) have increased significantly over the past four years. Today's physicians are looking for the financial security that accompanies an employed practice arrangement. Hospitals may represent a stable source of employment for these physicians. Physicians may be willing to sacrifice their autonomy for an employed position for many reasons (e.g., medical school loan indebtedness, high malpractice rates, high overhead costs associated with private practice, reimbursement struggles with insurers, time-consuming administration responsibilities). Due to current Stark regulations, it is also easier for hospitals to provide assistance to physicians when they are employees, although Stark III may make it easier for physicians in private practice to collaborate with hospitals.

The hospital-employed model has several ramifications for both hospitalist programs and the sponsoring hospital. This arrangement provides the hospitalist practice with the subsidy and financial security it needs to stay afloat. It provides the hospital with an inpatient program that it can market to both the existing medical staff and community, thereby potentially increasing market share for the hospital. Additionally, the hospital can market the program to potential primary care and/or specialist candidates who are considering relocation to the area (or for recruits fresh out of residency). Hospitalist support and an ongoing marketing program by the sponsoring hospital signify job security for hospitalist providers. Hospital-owned programs also provide value to their institutions by sharing a similar mission, vision, and objective.

According to Merritt, Hawkins and Associates, from April 1, 2007 to March 31, 2008, family medicine and internal medicine were the two most requested physician search assignments, followed by hospitalists. This is not surprising, considering the current shortage of primary care physicians, exacerbated by the increase in the aging and general population and the great demand for hospitalists (see Chapter 1). With ever-increasing frequency, established primary care and specialist physicians within a community are becoming hospital employees. Hospital-employed PCPs typically give up hospital medicine to focus on the outpatient practice setting. Many specialists, whether or not hospital employed, give up daily management of the patient and serve as consultants and/or *procedurists*: physicians who dedicate the majority of their time to performing various procedures in their field of expertise. The dynamics regarding these trends were discussed in Chapter I. Inpatient management of these patients is assumed by the hospitalist program. The physician-employed model (with hospitalist program utilization) can serve as an excellent tool to stabilize and grow a medical community. This phenomenon can also present a financial opportunity for the hospitalist program.

7.8 ASSESSMENT OF FAIR MARKET VALUE AND PHYSICIAN COMPENSATION

Most hospitalist programs will need to determine fair market value in order to establish appropriate physician compensation. There are several factors to consider in the valuation process. Program ownership (e.g., private, hospital owned, national management company) and tax status (e.g., for profit, tax exempt) will guide this process. The answers to these questions will determine if your program is affected directly by Stark regulations, antitrust laws, and concerns regarding gain sharing. In general, if your program is privately owned, compensation may be guided by your budget allowance (with marketplace guidance). If a subsidy is required from the sponsoring hospital for physician compensation, fair market value should be established. If your program performs a fair marketplace valuation, the following factors must all be considered. The weight of each factor will depend on the specific circumstances of your program.

Hospitalist Program Characteristics

Determination of hospitalist compensation will be guided by the focus of your program. For example, compensation will vary according to the patient population treated. Physicians who provide care for adults tend to receive greater compensation than those who treat pediatric inpatients exclusively. Traditional hospitalists tend to be more highly compensated than academicians. The reasons for these disparities in compensation are covered elsewhere in the book.

Physician Training

If providers have additional training (e.g., subspecialists) and/or skills, compensation may be greater than the marketplace average. Professional experience may also have a bearing on compensation. For example, in the open market, experienced hospitalists may command more than new graduates. Physicians in private practice (looking to transition to a hospitalist role) who are well known in the community may command greater compensation than an unknown candidate. If a candidate has administrative or leadership experience (e.g., as a clinical, quality assurance, or administrative director), this may also have a bearing on compensation.

Workload and Scope of Service

Physician workload and program scope of service will also influence compensation. For example, physicians who are expected to maintain a census of 20 patients per day tend to make more money than those who care for 10 to 12 patients each day. Programs providing 24/7 in-house coverage tend to compensate their physicians at higher levels for this service. Hospitalists who manage the hospital's observation or LTAC unit may also enjoy greater compensation. Finally, a clinical director hired to rejuvenate a failing program may be enticed by the compensation package. These are some examples that may warrant compensation above the fair market value.

Geography

Compensation will also be influenced by geographic considerations. For example, fair market value will be affected by hospitalist compensation in competing programs in the local community. Furthermore, fair compensation may be valuated regionally (e.g., North, South, East, West, Midwest) and by community size (e.g., rural, suburban, urban). Fair market valuations typically utilize data gathered by surveys (e.g., SHM biennual survey; MGMA; Merritt, Hawkins; *Today's Hospitalist*) specific for the specialty and job opportunity. Consultants may also be beneficial in establishing fair market compensation for your program.

Local and/or Extenuating Factors

There are other considerations in the compensation valuation process. For example, if there is fierce competition from local hospitalist programs in your community, you may decide to offer a compensation package that is significantly above fair market value. Furthermore, if your program experiences recruitment difficulties, this may warrant a compensation package that is greater than fair market value. Finally, if the hospitalist referral network (or specialist network) is destabilizing due to lack of program access for their patients, your program or the sponsoring hospital may need to hire another hospitalist immediately to remedy the situation. Recruitment in this circumstance may obviate physician compensation above fair market value.

Ultimately, establishing fair market compensation for your hospitalist physicians may involve a multitude of factors. These factors will be program specific and may or may not require legal counsel relating to Stark regulations or antitrust laws. Marketplace factors should only *guide* hospitalist compensation. There may be extenuating circumstances within your program that warrant physician compensation above and beyond what the market calls for.

8 Retention Initiatives

In the not too distant past, physicians entered the workforce immediately following residency and practiced in the same community for their entire career. Today, physicians are more mobile and don't hesitate to leave a practice and/or community several times during the course of their career. This is due in large part to generational factors (see Chapter 1). As a consequence, hospitalist programs must craft creative retention strategies addressing the core values and expectations of these physicians.

Employee turnover is costly for any organization. This is particularly true for physician practices. If a physician leaves a practice, there is typically an extended period of time (during recruitment) when the practice will be understaffed. This may lead to program instability and overworked hospitalists. The end result may be suboptimal physician performance and further job dissatisfaction.

Insufficient staffing during physician turnover may also lead to physician burnout and turnover of additional hospitalist providers. Numerous costs are associated with replacement of these doctors. These include costs associated with recruitment (e.g., headhunter fees, travel and lodging costs, sign-on bonuses, relocation expenses, medical school loan repayment, lost productivity for physician and nonphysician staff participating in the recruitment process), practice coverage (e.g., locum tenens), and lost revenues during provider shortages. Consequently, it is imperative that your program design a retention plan that minimizes physician turnover.

Before moving on, it's worth noting that not all turnover is detrimental. For example, a program can become more effective when performing poorly or when disruptive physicians depart. In addition, new physicians may bring both new ideas and skill sets to the program.

Hospitalist Recruitment and Retention: Building a Hospital Medicine Program,
By Kenneth G. Simone
Copyright © 2010 Wiley-Blackwell

They may also possess a high level of enthusiasm, which can be contagious and invigorate a practice.

Various retention initiatives have been discussed in previous chapters. In this chapter we briefly tie them together. We also discuss the creation of orientation and mentoring programs. An understanding of retention initiatives requires an appreciation for why physicians leave their jobs. Exhibit 8.1 lists some of the common reasons that hospitalists may leave a program, and Exhibit 8.2 lists the career choice of these departing hospitalists. Although Exhibit 8.1 is not all-inclusive, it highlights significant areas for focus when designing your retention plan. Programs should also be aware that employees strive for community, purpose, growth as a human being, growth as a professional, sense of personal impact, autonomy, and empowerment. Opportunities that can provide these will support physician retention.

Exhibit 8.1   Common Reasons That Physicians Leave Their Jobs

Physicians may leave their current practice for many reasons. The following are some of the more common reasons.

- Insufficient pay and/or benefits
- Unmet expectations
- Poor cultural fit with the practice or hospital (e.g., provider–practice mismatch)
- Poor fit within the community
- Spousal/significant other, family dissatisfaction with the community
- Lack of opportunities for career growth and advancement
- Inadequate support from practice or hospital (clinical and/or operational)
- Problems with practice clinical director or hospital administration
- Lack of work–life balance
- Lack of recognition
- Burnout

Exhibit 8.2   The Career Choice of Departing Hospitalists

The following information, the destination for hospitalists leaving their current practice, was obtained from the 2007–2008 SHM biennual survey.

- Another hospitalist program: 33%
- Fellowship/other training programs: 26%
- Different field of medicine: 22%
- Family/personal reasons: 9%
- Medical administration/consulting: 4%
- Retirement: 1%
- Other choice: 2%
- Unknown choice: 3%

8.1   DEFINING EXPECTATIONS AND FINDING THE APPROPRIATE FIT

Nearly one-half of all healthcare workers consider leaving their jobs within the first six months of employment! According to the 2006 American Medical Group Association (AMGA) and Cejka Search retention survey, the first three years in practice hold the greatest likelihood for turnover. Twelve percent leave within the first year, 46% within the first three years, and 23% after 10 years. Unmet expectations and poor cultural fit within the practice and/or community (including family members) may explain this early turnover.

The risk of physician turnover early in their employment underscores the importance of setting clear expectations with the candidate during the recruitment process. Recruiting programs must provide realistic details about the culture of the practice, hospital, and integrated healthcare delivery system. Expectations regarding physician workload, compensation, clinical performance, and nonclinical responsibilities must also be shared. The long-term vision and goals of the practice should be discussed and feedback should be sought regarding the candidate's expectations and vision. The recruitment team must then evaluate objectively if the candidate and program objectives are closely aligned. Selection of the ideal physician will support retention and minimize turnover within your practice.

8.2   WORK–LIFE BALANCE

Hospitalist programs should create a practice model and work schedule that support quality of life (e.g., flexible schedule, no call) for its physicians. Effective schedules offer physicians a work–life balance while maintaining both efficiency and continuity of care. Physician staffing and workload should be reasonable to ensure productivity but prevent burnout. Creation of a staffing plan for periods when the practice is short-staffed (in the event of physician turnover or illness) will support the goals of workload balance and high-quality patient care. If your program succeeds at this challenge, hospitalist retention will be supported.

8.3   INTEGRATION OF THE HOSPITALIST PROGRAM AND HOSPITALIST PHYSICIANS

Strategies promoting and supporting hospitalist physicians within the medical staff and hospital staff will also be a valuable retention tool. This can be accomplished by providing both quarterly hospitalist program updates (via a hospitalist newsletter) and an annual presentation to both the medical and hospital staff. The hospitalists may also offer educational programs for the medical staff and/or hospital staff. These educational programs include nursing staff in-service training, ACLS training, code blue training, and rapid-response team training, to name a few examples. The physicians can also integrate themselves within the medical staff by serving on key medical staff committees and/or serving in medical staff leadership positions. Finally, some hospitalist programs allow their physicians to become involved in teaching residents and medical students or working in a specialty clinic as a means of supporting job satisfaction and retention within the practice.

8.4   SUPPORT FROM THE CLINICAL DIRECTOR AND SPONSORING HOSPITAL

A hospitalist clinical director and hospitalist administrator who is supportive and attentive to a new physician's needs is invaluable in the retention process. It is widely known that many employees leave their job when they have trouble with their supervisor. Therefore, it is prudent to provide the clinical director with the support that he or she needs to be an effective supervisor. Effective supervisors must be clear in their expectations and provide constructive criticism. They should offer encouragement and assist in professional development and growth. In addition, they must keep the staff informed, encouraging input and feedback from them, and treating all staff fairly. Finally, the director should meet with new physicians at one, three, and six months following the date of hire. During these meetings the director should obtain feedback from the new doctor as well as review performance.

Hospitalist administrators (and hospital administration) must also be excellent communicators and must be approachable. They should inspire trust and confidence within the organization. There should be transparency between the sponsoring hospital and hospitalist practice. Policies regarding regular hospitalist practice meetings and meetings with hospital administration should be created to bolster support for the hospitalists and provide a forum for discussion. Some programs also hold an annual hospitalist–hospital weekend retreat (a valuable team building tool).

8.5   CLINICAL AND OPERATIONAL SUPPORT

Hospitalist programs and their sponsoring institutions can develop operational tactics that support practice objectives, clinical excellence, and physician retention. These include, for example, the development of interdisciplinary morning rounds, a case management program, and a pharmacy consultation service. In addition, a hospitalist performance scorecard and committee can be created to monitor physician performance and provide feedback. Concurrent core measure performance review will also be beneficial. Utilization of a standardized communication system (e.g., EMR, voice mail, PDA) is another example of a supportive tactic. There are many other initiatives that may be employed. Although development of all these tactics may appear ambitious, they can be created with time. Refer to Section 11.6 for a detailed discussion on operational tactics and collaborative systems of care.

8.6   OPPORTUNITIES FOR CAREER GROWTH AND ADVANCEMENT

Creation of an ongoing educational series for the hospitalist physicians supports both performance and job satisfaction. These educational initiatives may address coding and chart documentation, medicolegal risk, pay-for-performance and core measure expectations, customer service, communication techniques, and conflict management and resolution. These are all areas that are germane to the day-to-day hospitalist activities.

Hospitalist programs that provide for physician growth and/or professional advancement support retention. For example, the program may fund educational courses that foster development of new clinical skills (e.g., procedural) or leadership skills that the physician can bring back and utilize in his or her current program. These educational initiatives may include development of administrative (e.g., executive) and business skills as well. The sponsoring hospital may develop a leadership tract within the institution to groom potential (hospitalist) medical staff leaders. In this way the hospitalist program and sponsoring hospital support physician growth by offering diverse opportunities and challenges leading to both professional and job satisfaction.

8.7 FINANCIAL OPPORTUNITIES

Creation of an incentive plan can provide a win–win result for both practice and physician and is another effective retention strategy. The incentive plan allows the hospitalist to be positively recognized and rewarded financially for his or her performance. It also benefits the hospital by enhancing the quality of care. Some hospitalist practices provide incentives for the creation of additional hospitalist services and/or clinical programs, thus adding another benefit for the hospital. Incentive programs also empower physicians by allowing some control over income potential.

8.8 SPOUSAL/SIGNIFICANT OTHER AND FAMILY INTEGRATION WITHIN THE COMMUNITY

Retention strategies would not be complete without a discussion of initiatives involving the candidate's family. As stated in Chapter 5, community fit for spouse/significant other and family is an important factor influencing physician retention. Consequently, it is important to get spousal involvement in the recruitment process early on (e.g., recruiting the family will go a long way toward retaining the physician candidate). This recruitment initiative is discussed in Chapter 9. Once the newly hired physician and his or her family arrive in town, it is important to engage the family during initiation into the community. Successful integration of the new hospitalist's family into the community may ultimately influence physician retention. This can be coordinated with the mentor program. Suffice it to say that if the family is unhappy in a new location, it will be very difficult to keep the new physician happy.

8.9   THE ORIENTATION PROGRAM

The retention process begins formally on the first day of work (it begins unofficially with the initial contact between the program and candidate). A comprehensive orientation program will be beneficial for the new physician and support retention. Some practices dedicate three to five days for orientation and job shadowing. Although this may appear to be a prolonged time dedicated to orientation, the payback (e.g., retention) is priceless. The program's clinical director and practice manager (if one exists) should coordinate the process. Exhibit 8.3 lists the common elements of an orientation program.

Although the program's specific policies, procedures, and protocols may have been discussed in the recruitment phase, the orientation period is a time to present this information in detail and reinforce its importance. It is also important to present the history of the program along with its mission and objectives so that the new physician will have a clear understanding of both the program's role and his or her contribution. A practice policy and procedures manual should be provided during this orientation period. This manual should be reviewed in detail and signed-off on by the new hire, indicating that all the information was covered.

The hospitalist clinical director should review the job description and clinical expectations with the physician early in the orientation process. As with the policy and procedures manual, provide a copy to the new physician and have him or her sign off. It's also beneficial to discuss medical record documentation standards. A copy of all hospitalist pre-printed order sheets and clinical guidelines can be provided at this time. The clinical aspects of the incentive plan can be discussed as well.

Discuss the hospitalist practice model and its key operating principles. This includes discussion of provider schedules, the various shifts that exist (e.g., day, swing, float, backup, night), the presence or absence of weekend and/or night call, and holiday call responsibilities. Vacation time, CME time, and sick time should be addressed as well. Share the protocol for moonlighting (in-house or at other institutions) if it is allowed by your program.

Discussion of hospitalist communication standards is prudent during orientation. This involves a review of the communication modalities (e.g., Internet, fax, voice mail, telephone, PDA) utilized by the practice. It also includes detailed discussion of the morning, evening, weekend, and holiday sign-out protocol. The procedure for morning

Exhibit 8.3   Orientation Protocol

A robust orientation program covers a diverse set of subjects and involves the accomplishment of numerous tasks. The goal of this program is to support both the success and the long-term retention of the new physician. Following is an example of such a program.

1. Specific topics to be discussed with the new physician include:
   - Review history, mission, values, and objectives of the program
   - Review mission, values, and objectives of the hospital (if hospital employed)
   - Review practice policy and procedure manual
   - Review job description
   - Review incentive plan
   - Review medical record documentation standards
   - Review practice model and key operating principles
   - Review medical staff roster
   - Review professional relationships in the community
   - Review communication standards
   - Review hospital medical record/EMR system
2. Provide coding and medical record documentation educational sessions.
3. Assign a mentor.
4. Tour the facilities.
5. Tour the key referral offices (meet and greet).
6. Tour various hospital departments: meet and greet (e.g., nursing, imaging, cardiopulmonary, social service, case management, pharmacy).
7. Meet with the hospital administrator overseeing the hospitalist program.
8. Job-shadow other hospitalists (possibly the mentor).
9. Organize a "welcome reception" with the medical community and hospital staff.
10. Place an announcement in the local newspaper welcoming the new physician into the community.
11. Print business cards for the new hospitalist.
12. Update both the practice the web site and the brochure (including a picture and biography of the new hospitalist).

rounds should be reviewed. Additional topics include the hand-off process between referring provider and hospitalist (at admission and discharge), and among hospitalist providers (with transfer of attending care). Communication protocols should also be addressed between hospitalist and specialist, and between the patient/family and the hospitalist provider. Review the EMR (if one exists) and organization of the hospital medical record in detail. Information Technology (IT) sessions are highly recommended for computer/EMR training.

Review of the medical staff roster and outpatient providers (and practice groups) in the community will be a helpful guide for the new physician. Distribute a roster of the providers participating with the hospitalist program (e.g., PCP and specialist referral network) as well as a list of preferred specialists. Highlight the established professional relationships in the community. A tour of the key referral offices will be valuable at this time and should be scheduled. This "meet and greet" initiative will break the ice for the new hospitalist and help all stake-holders put a face to a name. It is also an effective marketing and cus-tomer service tactic. This visit illustrates the emphasis that the hospitalist practice places on the referring provider–hospitalist relationship.

Tour the hospital facilities and visit various hospital departments. Spon-sor a "meet and greet" with the various stakeholders (e.g., nursing, imaging, cardiopulmonary, social service, case management, pharmacy). This can occur at a luncheon or an after-hours gathering. Meet with the hospital administrative team (including the administrator overseeing the program) as well, and establish an open and collaborative relationship early on.

Conducting educational sessions on coding and documentation is extremely valuable to both the physician and the practice (regardless of physician familiarity with coding). Typically, a coding specialist over-sees this initiative if your program (or the hospital) employs one. If one is not available, it is worthwhile to contract with a consultant to provide this service. During these sessions the new physician should be instructed in Evaluation and Management (E/M) and ICD-9 coding guidelines. He or she should also be educated regarding appropriate medical record documentation. If your program uses progress note templates, review them at this time. Finally, instruct the physician on the appropriate billing protocol. These instructional sessions will be money well spent, as they will provide the practice with the potential for greater income through appropriate coding. Add the additional benefit of reducing medicolegal risk (with appropriate medical record documentation) and this initiative is invaluable.

Assigning a mentor is another valuable tool of retention. A hospitalist mentor is well positioned to provide the new employee with information and insight regarding the medical staff, hospital staff, hospital administration, medical community at large, hospitalist practice, and community. The new physician can also job shadow this person for the first few days of clinical work. The ideal mentor should be someone who shares similar age, personality, ethnical background, work style, interests/hobbies, or family circumstances (e.g., children of the same age) with the new physician. This person can ease the transition of the new employee into his or her role as hospitalist. Regular contact should be maintained with the new physician for at least the first six to 12 months. During these designated times the mentor should check in on the physician's well-being and to ensure that there are no major problems (professional/social) or workplace obstacles. The mentor and his or her family can also serve as an excellent resource for the new employee's family.

8.10   THE EXIT INTERVIEW

Conducting an exit interview with the departing physician can provide valuable information. The objective of this interview is to obtain honest feedback from the physician regarding the hospitalist practice, hospital, community, and his or her reasons for leaving. For example, information can be obtained concerning the effectiveness of the clinical director, the culture of the practice, as well as the strengths and weaknesses of the program. In addition, information may be provided pertaining to the strengths, weaknesses, and culture of both the hospital and community. The information gleaned from the exit interview can be applied to solve problems that may exist within the practice. In this way the exit interview serves as an excellent retention tactic for future employees.

The exit interview can be performed by the human resource director if your program employs one or by an objective third party. It will be most effective if it is done prior to the physician's departure or shortly thereafter. The interview should be performed in a private area to ensure confidentiality. The interviewer should listen carefully, avoid making assumptions, and avoid engaging the person in an argument.

It is best to save the hardest questions for the latter part of the interview. If the practice is willing to serve as a reference (e.g., recommend the physician), it may be helpful to make that offer at the onset of the interview. Query the departing physician regarding suggestions to improve the practice. Obtain his or her perspective regarding the compensation and benefit package. The practice should also determine and document if it would rehire the physician. A sample of exit interview questions is provided in Exhibit 8.4.

Exhibit 8.4   Exit Interview Questions

Various formats can be used for exit interview questions to obtain the desired information. Utilizing a combination of open-ended questions and questions with a rating system can be an effective method.

- What triggered your decision to leave the practice?
- Rate the following (1, excellent; 2, very good; 3, good; 4, average; 5, poor; 6, unacceptable) and explain why.
  - Practice scope of service and objectives
  - Hospitalist orientation program
  - Practice model and provider schedule (including call)
  - Daily workload
  - Cooperation within the practice
  - Communication within the practice
  - Communication within the organization as a whole
  - Practice policies and procedures
  - Clinical director support and quality of supervision
  - Hospitalist (nonclinical) staff support
  - Hospitalist administrator support
  - Sponsoring institution support
  - Hospital services and support staff
  - Medical staff availability and support
  - Ability for professional growth and development
  - Compensation and benefits
  - Family satisfaction with the community
- Evaluate the hospitalist clinical director (1, excellent; 2, very good; 3, good; 4, average; 5, poor; 6, unacceptable) in regard to the following:
  - Demonstrated fair and equal treatment with all hospitalist physicians
  - Resolved physician complaints and problems (and in a timely manner)
  - Consistently followed practice policies and procedures
  - Provided regular feedback and job recognition
  - Provided annual performance reviews and did so in a constructive manner
  - Led by example and was a positive influence

- ○ Demonstrated effective leadership qualities fostering cooperation and teamwork
- ○ Encouraged and valued feedback
- Did you understand the job expectations when you were hired?
- Did you receive sufficient training to meet those expectations?
- Were you aware of the program's mission, vision, objectives, and values?
- Were you aware of the hospital's mission, vision, objectives, and values?
- What five things did you like best about the job?
- What five things did you like least about the job?
- What five things did you like most about the hospital?
- What five things did you like least about the hospital?
- Do you have suggestions to improve hospitalist work performance standards?
- Do you have suggestions to improve the operation and management of the practice?
- Would you be interested in staying if certain things changed? What would those be?
- Would you consider returning to the practice in the future?
- Would you recommend this practice to colleagues as a place of employment?
- What does your new employment offer that this practice could not?

9 Putting It All Together: The Site Visit and Interview

There are several factors to consider during the recruitment process, many of which have been discussed in previous chapters. For example, programs must have a handle on the hospitalist physician recruitment pool (e.g., the local and national marketplace) from which to build a network. In addition, the recruitment team must have common vision as to the potential hire (e.g., skills, training, experience). Programs must also develop a sourcing strategy (refer to Chapter 4 for a detailed discussion of sourcing). Finally, programs must decide who will participate on the recruitment team.

The recruitment team must be constructed carefully and each member's role defined clearly. Consider including the hospitalist administrator, clinical director, and practice manager as the core members of the recruitment team. Key contact information should flow through these persons. Other recruitment team participants may include additional hospitalists, the sponsoring hospital's CEO or COO, referring physicians (e.g., users of the program), specialists on the medical staff, the sponsoring hospital's medical staff coordinator, the hospital staff (e.g., director of nursing, case management director), key community leaders, and in some instances, hospital board members. The role of each member is defined later in the chapter.

When creating your recruitment plan, take into account where the current hospitalists in the practice have come from and what attracted them to the practice. For example, the candidate may be attracted to the hospitalist practice model, the call schedule, the practice philosophy and scope of service, the sponsoring hospital's facilities and resources, or the availability of medical and surgical specialists. The attraction may also revolve around family needs within the community,

Hospitalist Recruitment and Retention: Building a Hospital Medicine Program,
By Kenneth G. Simone
Copyright © 2010 Wiley-Blackwell

such as spousal/significant other (referred to simply as spousal for the duration of the chapter) career opportunities, educational opportunities for the children, geographic location, recreational/quality-of-life considerations (e.g., lakes/ocean, mountains, climate, culture, crime rate) or proximity to major cities and airlines. This information will be valuable when marketing the program to recruits and ultimately in finding a good match.

A hospitalist recruitment manual should be written choreographing the process in detail. The process can be divided into three phases: the contact, the site visit, and the postvisit phase. The objectives of each phase must be defined clearly and the execution must be well coordinated. Several responsibilities accompany each phase. Various recruitment team members will be involved at different stages in this process and must follow a logistical sequence.

Recruitment programs must never lose focus on what's at stake. There's enormous pressure on hospitalist programs to "get it right" the first time. Poor recruitment can have a number of adverse consequences for a hospitalist practice. As discussed previously, it may result in higher turnover rates, leading to practice instability. This, in turn, may lead to low staff morale, job dissatisfaction, and poor physician performance. This is an expensive proposition. Recruitment of a solid candidate can rejuvenate a failing program, instilling energy through new and progressive concepts, and support job satisfaction and program stability.

9.1   THE CONTACT

In all likelihood, hospitalist programs will receive curricula vitae (CVs) from many sources. The hospitalist practice manager or practice administrator (referred to as the recruitment coordinator for the duration of the chapter) should serve as the initial contact person. If the program utilizes a recruiter, the candidate will be prescreened to make sure that the opportunity is consistent with the candidate's professional and personal objectives. Upon receipt of a CV, distribute it to the person(s) responsible for initial screening. This is ordinarily performed by the hospitalist clinical director. The screener should assess the candidate's education, clinical training, skill sets, and professional work experience. Closely review the CV to ensure that there are no gaps in the professional timeline, inconsistent information, or ambiguous wording. Assess the timeline for frequent job changes, as this may indicate professional instability or other worrisome problems. If any questions arise, request clarification directly from the physician candidate.

If the candidate is deemed acceptable on paper, the clinical director should make telephone contact, preferably within five days of receipt of the CV. Provide as much information as possible about the practice opportunity while learning about the candidate's motivations. The goals of the telephone screen are twofold. The screener is accessing the candidate for the desired traits of the new physician and to assess the likelihood of the candidate's acceptance of the position. During this call, present the program's mission, vision, and objectives. Query the candidate regarding his or her professional interests, short- and long-term goals, and ambitions. Effective questioning will produce truthful responses without leading the candidate in a desired direction. Discuss the candidate's financial expectations and practice aspirations regarding scope of service, work schedule, workload, hospital size, and so on. Review his or her personal interests and lifestyle needs, addressing community preferences (e.g., location, size, culture, climate, schooling) and family considerations (e.g., occupational, educational, proximity to extended family). Learn as much as you can about the spouse's professional and personal interests as well. When physician candidates refuse an employment position, 60% of the time it is because of spousal dissatisfaction with factors related to the job opportunity. This underscores the need to make the spouse an integral part of the interview process (previsit and during the site visit).

If the screen is satisfactory, invite the candidate and spouse/family for a site visit and send a recruitment packet. All recruitment expenses, including airfare, lodging, meals, and transportation (e.g., car rental, taxi, train, shuttle), should be provided by your program (the candidate should assume all expenses if he or she extends the visit for personal reasons beyond the recruitment period). The recruitment packet should contain the hospitalist practice brochure (with Web site address), the hospitalist program recruitment video (if one exists), the sponsoring hospital's brochure/video, sample copies of medical staff newsletters, and materials regarding the chamber of commerce and other organizations (e.g., performing arts center, recreational and outdoor guide, dining guide, local theater, college systems). When creating the recruitment packet, consult with a public relations or marketing specialist for innovative concepts. Keep in mind that it's a buyer's market and that most hospitalist candidates have many job offers to consider. Creative marketing strategies that stand out may provide your program with an edge.

Contact the real estate agent as well. It is prudent for all programs to have an established relationship with an agent for just this purpose. In many cases the real estate agent assists in recruitment by actively selling the community (e.g., discussing school systems, neighborhoods, crime rate, millage rates/taxes, cost of living, cultural offerings). The agent should contact the candidate and spouse regarding housing specifications and transmit relevant information for review before the site visit. This will make the real estate tour more productive.

Obtain professional references before the site visit. Written permission should be granted by the candidate prior to contacting people listed as references. Contact current and previous clinical supervisors or directors. It may also be beneficial to contact the president of the medical staff and/or chief medical officer. If the candidate is a new graduate, contact the residency director and faculty advisor. The hospitalist clinical director should speak directly to these persons in addition to obtaining a written reference. Subtle cues may be provided by a reference via the telephone call that may not appear in writing.

Reference checks involve assessment of the candidate's clinical skills, judgment, competency, and work ethic. This includes the physician's ability to manage clinical resources appropriately and practice in a fiscally responsible manner. It also involves assessment of both the candidate's interpersonal and communication skills with practice associates, patients, colleagues, hospital staff, and administration (both practice and hospital if applicable). Other essential information includes appraisal of the person's leadership skills/potential and his or her ability to work within a team structure. Finally, it is extremely important to assess if the candidate is a positive or negative force within the current practice as well as his or her ability to deal with stress (including coping mechanisms).

In addition to clinical references, query the national data bank and state medical association, ensuring that there are no outstanding problems with lawsuits, license suspension, license restrictions, and the like. In addition, check with both the current employer and hospital regarding restrictions of clinical privileges and medical staff issues. Run both a criminal and a credit check, verify medical school graduation, and confirm specialty board certification. These steps can help prevent the fallout (e.g., practice dysfunction) associated with a bad hire. In addition, these steps can save your program from the many costs associated with recruitment (including the site visit), as well as the embarrassment associated with making a significant hiring error.

9.2 THE SITE VISIT

The recruitment coordinator must create an itinerary for the site visit. The dates should be coordinated so that all key participants are available. Participants may vary, depending on the particular candidate. For example, if a community physician attended the same medical school or residency training program as the candidate, he or she should be invited to attend the recruitment dinner. If the candidate's spouse is a banker, invite the board member who is president of the local bank to a reception and/or recruitment dinner. Allot three days for the site visit if possible (e.g., depending on the candidate's schedule and time restrictions). This will allow time for the candidate and his or her family to explore the community.

The recruitment team must be sensitive to the needs of the candidate's family during the evaluation process. Make the spouse an integral part of the interview process. Remember, your program must appeal to both the family and the candidate. In some circumstances it may be productive to prepare a separate itinerary for the candidate's spouse (see Exhibit 9.1). This may include interviews with potential employers, churches, schools, and the like. It may also include a visit to the local museum, zoo, or park if children are present. Pairing the candidate's spouse/family with another spouse/family (matched by common interests, life circumstances, etc.) during the visit can be valuable.

Closely coordinate the site visit arrangements with the candidate. This includes flight reservations, transportation from and to the airport (e.g., pickup or car rental), lodging accommodations, and directions to the hotel and hospital. Other arrangements include coordination of the tours (of the hospitalist practice, hospital, and referring physician's offices), activities for the spouse (and children, if applicable), as well as lunch and dinner reservations. The recruitment coordinator should serve as the contact or "go to" person for the physician. The candidate can contact this person with any questions and needs that may arise at any time following the telephone screen through the site visit and return home. The real estate and community tour should be coordinated with the real estate agent in conjunction with the candidate and practice coordinator.

The recruitment coordinator is responsible for distributing the itinerary and candidate's CV to all key participants in the recruitment process. All participants should familiarize themselves with this information. The coordinator must also make sure that the candidate stays on schedule and is where he or she should be at all times. A

Exhibit 9.1   The Spouse/Family Site Visit Itinerary

Create a site visit itinerary for the spouse and family (while the candidate tours the facilities and meets with the various stakeholders) if the circumstances allow. The choice of guide will vary depending on the specific circumstances and interests of the spouse/family. Utilizing a guide who shares common interests, life circumstances, or a similar profession will be valuable. The following is a generic itinerary:

- Guide to pick up spouse/family at the hotel
- Breakfast
- Meet with potential business contacts and/or employers at businesses of interest (to interview and/or discuss professional opportunities)
- Lunch
- Visit schools of interest and meet with school principal and/or visit and tour local colleges
- Visit various churches, synagogues, and mosques, and meet with representatives
- Visit museums and park if appropriate

---

contingency plan should be in place for unexpected last-minute changes. An example of a site visit itinerary with a description of participant responsibilities is presented in Exhibit 9.2.

Participation of various medical and hospital staff members is an excellent recruitment tool, as it demonstrates support (by these key stakeholders) for the program. Provide the recruitment team members with talking points to guide them and to ensure that all relevant material is covered with the candidate (see Exhibit 9.3). Conversely, allow the candidate time to discuss topics of concern or of great interest to him or her. The team must not get so caught up in the process that they lose focus on the candidate.

Encourage all participants to be truthful with the candidate. Coach your team to accomplish this in a constructive and positive manner. You do not want a person casting a negative light on the practice or being perceived as a negative force. Your program may lose an excellent candidate as a result. Candidates do not want to work in a negative or hostile environment.

Exhibit 9.2   Site Visit Itinerary

The following is a sample itinerary that can be modified to meet your program's needs. The specifics will depend on the candidate's specifics (e.g., training, professional interests, marital status, occupation of spouse, children, hobbies) and the availability of key participants. Clearly define each participant's role and objectives in the recruitment process. Develop a protocol to collect and assimilate the information in a timely manner.

- *Day 1*
  - Arrange for pickup of candidate at airport or for car rental
  - Arrange for a card and fruit basket or floral arrangement welcoming the candidate at the hotel room
- *Day 2*
  - Clinical director to pick up or meet and greet candidate at the hospitalist practice office
  - Introduction and breakfast with the hospitalists and nonclinician staff
  - Hospitalist office tour
  - Hospital tour, on which various department chiefs (e.g., physicians) and managers are introduced:
    - ED
    - Nursing director and department supervisors
    - Diagnostic imaging
    - Cardiopulmonary
    - Laboratory/pathology
    - Surgery
    - Social service
    - Case management
    - Pharmacy
    - Medical records
  - Job shadow on hospital units (optional)
  - Interview with hospitalist clinical director
  - Interview with hospitalist administrator
  - Lunch with hospitalists, various hospital medical staff, and community PCPs (e.g., referring physicians)
  - Interview with hospital CEO/COO (if hospital-owned practice)

- ○ Meet with hospital quality assurance director (optional)
- ○ Meet with chief medical officer of the hospital (or vice president of medical affairs)
- ○ Meet with the medical staff president (optional)
- ○ Meet and greet tour of select referring PCP offices (optional)
- ○ Reception with hospital staff and hospital administration
- ○ Dinner with family (participants may be selected from the following: the hospitalist clinical director and other hospitalist physicians, referring PCPs, specialists, key hospital board members, key community leaders, etc.)
- • *Day 3: Community tour*
  - ○ Various neighborhoods
  - ○ Local schools and churches, synagogues, or mosques)
  - ○ College campuses
  - ○ Performing arts center
  - ○ Shopping malls
  - ○ Downtown district
  - ○ Famous landmarks
  - ○ Waterfront (e.g., ocean, lakes) and/or mountains, if applicable
- • *Free time/departure:* recommend day trips (if the candidate is staying longer)

N.B.: Consider scheduling a visit with a mortgage loan officer to assist the candidate in securing a home loan.

Exhibit 9.3   Recruitment Talking Points

The following are examples of talking points that your program should consider discussing with the candidate:

- • Historical overview of the practice (including mission, vision, and objectives)
- • Relationship with sponsoring hospital
- • Schedule specifics
  - ○ Practice model
  - ○ Staffing numbers and provider type (e.g., IM, FP, IM/pediatrics, pediatrics, NPC)

- ◦ Daytime and nighttime hours
- ◦ Call, weekend responsibilities, holiday responsibilities, schedule flexibility, and so on
- Job description
- Hospitalist program responsibilities
  - ◦ Hospital coverage (e.g., 7 a.m. to 7 p.m., 24/7 in-house, etc.)
  - ◦ Unassigned ED call
  - ◦ Surgical co-management
  - ◦ Rapid-response team participation
  - ◦ Code blue coverage
  - ◦ Palliative care service
  - ◦ Observation unit management
  - ◦ LTAC unit management
  - ◦ Preoperative clinic
  - ◦ Oversight of quality and patient safety initiatives
  - ◦ Committee work
  - ◦ Residency program
- Inquire about the candidate's specific practice expectations and medical experience
- Practice utilization
  - ◦ ADC
  - ◦ Number of admissions and discharges per year by practice and provider
  - ◦ Number of consultations per year by practice and provider
- Referral base, referral patterns
  - ◦ Specific practices/specific providers
  - ◦ Specific hospitals (e.g., rural hospital transfers)
  - ◦ Geographic range
  - ◦ Professional relationships
- Patient mix (e.g., by diagnostic related group)
- Payor mix
- Availability of hospitalist support staff (e.g., office manager, secretary, medical assistant)
- Practice facilities and equipment
  - ◦ Office space (e.g., dedicated workstations)
  - ◦ Call room
  - ◦ Practice resources (e.g., library, online resources, PDA, laptop)

- Discuss program operational and organizational chain of command
- Medical staff support (e.g., availability of specific specialties)
  - Review hospital medical staff roster composition
  - Open vs. closed medical staff; discuss specialties available in the community not offered at the hospital
- Hospital support staff
  - Nursing expertise
  - Case management
  - ED
  - Utilization review and social service
  - Pharmacy department
  - Physical therapy/Occupational therapy department
  - Home health and hospice
  - Rapid-response team
- Discuss hospital resources and programs, including hospitalist case management program, interdisciplinary morning hospital rounds with the hospitalists, home health and hospice, outpatient infusion department, congestive heart failure (CHF) clinic, and so on
- Discuss procedures and services provided at the hospital
  - Cardiac catherization lab (diagnostic vs. interventional)
  - Surgical services (e.g., coronary artery bypass graft, transplants, neurosurgery)
  - Interventional radiology
  - Vascular services, lithotripsy, bronchoscope, hyperbaric chamber, wound clinic, burn unit, and so on
  - Intensivist service (open vs. closed ICU/critical care unit)
  - Technological resources
    - Sixty-four-slice CT scan
    - MRI
    - PET scan
    - Computer physician order entry (CPOE), electronic medical record (EMR)
    - Data tracking systems for clinical performance, financial performance, and resource utilization
- Discuss procedures and services offered within the community but not at the hospital; for example:
  - Open heart program
  - Interventional cardiac catherization lab

- ○ Dialysis unit
- ○ Radiation oncology
- Relationship with the community
- Local healthcare climate and politics
  - ○ Number of hospitals in the community
  - ○ Number of hospitalist programs in the community
  - ○ Geographic location of the closest tertiary care centers
  - ○ Geographic location of centers of excellence
  - ○ Local medicolegal landscape
- Income opportunity
  - ○ Salary, benefits, incentive plan, profit share
  - ○ Vacation and CME time
  - ○ Sign-on bonus, school loan repayment, relocation stipend, and so on
- Practice ownership (e.g., hospital, multispecialty group, hospitalist only)
- Opportunity for practice partnership (e.g., private group)
- Opportunities for practice growth (e.g., develop new programs such as a hospitalist-managed observation unit, palliative care service, preop clinic)
- Opportunity for career growth
  - ○ Teaching
  - ○ Research
  - ○ Leadership appointments, medical directorships, and so on
  - ○ Administrative
  - ○ Participation in specialty clinics
- Discuss specifics about the community, including:
  - ○ Neighborhoods (e.g., location, affordability of housing, safety, tax rate)
  - ○ School system/local colleges
  - ○ Major industries
  - ○ Culture (e.g., demographics and cultural mix)
  - ○ Recreational activities
  - ○ Dining and entertainment
  - ○ Spiritual resources (churches)
  - ○ Potential work contacts for spouse

9.3   THE RECRUITMENT TEAM

Next, we examine some recommendations regarding the composition and role of the recruitment team.

Clinical Director

The clinical director is the principal source of clinical and operational information. Discussion topics include the program's mission, vision, objectives, policies and procedures, practice model, and call schedule. The director will interview the candidate and play a supportive role from the first telephone contact with the candidate through the decision-making process (and beyond if the physician is hired).

The clinical director should discuss the strengths and weaknesses of the program, sharing the corrective action plan in place to address each weakness. The program's short- and long-term strategic plan can be discussed briefly at this time. The existence of a strategic plan conveys the fact that your program has organizational stability, leadership oversight, and is sustainable. Program stability will support your recruitment efforts.

The clinical director must review the job description with the candidate. See Exhibit 9.4 for a sample hospitalist job description. Create a job overview to complement the job description. It will provide the candidate with a realistic description of both the expectations and responsibilities of the position. Include a description of the typical workday, addressing the number of work hours each day, ADC per physician, as well as the average number of admissions, consultations, and discharges per physician each day. Share aspects of the job that are both rewarding and challenging. Take time to mention support systems that are in place to assist the physician. Discuss opportunities

---

Exhibit 9.4   Hospitalist Job Description

Create the hospitalist job description based on the expectations and responsibilities of your program. These expectations and responsibilities vary from program to program depending on its mission, objectives, and scope of service. In general, the job description should address several areas.

- *Position summary.* Provide a brief description of the job responsibilities. For example, the summary may state that the hospitalist provides patient care to hospitalized patients (utilizing evidence-based clinical guidelines and adhering to quality/patient safety initiatives), provides clinical supervision of NPCs, and supports the mission, values, and objectives of the hospitalist program (and hospital if employed by the hospital). It may also state that the physician is responsible for adhering to the program's policies, procedures, and strategic plan.

- *Essential job functions*
  - Clinical responsibilities
  - Administrative responsibilities
- *Supervisory responsibilities.* If your hospitalist program requires hospitalist supervision of NPCs, residents/interns, or medical students, this should be stated clearly.
- *Reporting structure.* State clearly who reports to the physician and to whom the physician reports.
- *Job requirements and expectations.* Define clearly hospitalist requirements and expectations. For example, he or she must:
  - Have an unrestricted medical license to practice medicine in the state or states where your program is located
  - Be credentialed and privileged to practice medicine at the sponsoring hospital
  - Work whatever the number of hours per week and the number of call hours per week required by your program (if your program has call responsibilities)
  - Provide necessary administrative time each week to complete medical records (as consistent with medical staff bylaw requirements) and all paperwork in a timely manner
  - Complete the specified number of CME hours (annually or biennually) as required by the medical staff bylaws and state licensure board
- *Knowledge, skills, and abilities required.* Address the core competencies that a hospitalist physician must possess in your program. This should include:
  - The ability to develop treatment plans, manage patients, and develop discharge plans for each patient
  - The ability to establish and maintain strong line of communication with key stakeholders (e.g., patients/families, referring PCPs, specialists, nurses, hospital administration)
  - Possessing in-depth coding and chart documentation knowledge
  - Possessing knowledge of both the hospitalist and the integrated healthcare delivery network system

- ○ The ability to demonstrate strong analytical skills regarding appropriate resource utilization
- ○ The ability to participate in the development of evidence-based clinical protocols
- ○ The ability to analyze data and assess clinical performance as it relates to quality care and clinical outcomes
- ○ Possessing skill in establishing and maintaining effective and collaborative working relationships with the medical staff, referring providers, hospital staff, and the community
- ○ The ability to supervise NPCs, residents, interns, and medical students (if applicable)

- *Typical working conditions.* Describe the typical work environment (both office and hospital) and discuss potential exposures (e.g., communicable diseases, toxic substances, medicinal preparations, needles, body fluids)
- *Typical physical demands.* Describe the typical physical activities and skills required (e.g., sitting, standing, reaching, lifting patients with assistance, normal range of hearing and eyesight, hand–eye coordination, manual dexterity to operate computer keyboard and telephone)
- *Education and work experience required.* Address the following:
  - ○ Work experience required (e.g., three to five years as a practicing hospitalist or in private practice)
  - ○ Educational experience required (e.g., must be a graduate of an accredited allopathic/osteopathic medical school)
  - ○ Training experience required [e.g., must complete an internal medicine, family practice, or medicine–pediatrics residency (if an adult program) or a pediatric residency (if a pediatric program)]
  - ○ Board certification requirements (e.g., must be board certified or board eligible; if a board exam hasn't been completed, require certification within two years)
  - ○ Reference requirements (e.g., must have acceptable references from the director of the residency training program, physicians, hospital personnel, previous employers, and persons chosen by your program; (references are difficult to assess for a number of reasons, and it may be beneficial in some instances to choose the reference)

for advancement and professional development. This preemptive strategy will help screen out physicians who are a poor match for your program. It may also reduce unrealistic expectations on the part of the candidate, enhancing both job satisfaction and performance while reducing turnover for those physicians who choose your program.

Hospitalist Administrator

The hospitalist administrator's role is to review the nonclinical administrative duties, reinforce the practice mission, vision, values, and objectives, and discuss contract parameters (including a "ballpark" salary range, number of work hours per week, benefits, vacation time, CME time, etc.). The administrator will serve as the go-to person for contractual and logistical issues.

Hospitalist Physicians

Hospitalists within the practice should provide a realistic perspective of the program and sponsoring hospital. They can serve as a peer resource for the candidate. Choose those physicians who are excellent communicators and who have a positive point of view.

Sponsoring Hospital's CEO or COO

The hospital administrator will provide information pertaining to the hospital's' mission, vision, and objectives. He or she should review the hospital's current service line and discuss the short- and long-term plans for the hospital. The administrator should share his or her perspective of the hospitalist program and elaborate on the program's role and significance in the hospital's future.

Referring Physicians

Referring physicians will provide a perspective on the outpatient provider's needs and expectations regarding the hospitalist program. They should discuss their level of satisfaction with the program and communicate support for the program. Furthermore, they can share how the program has affected their quality of life.

Specialists

Specialists will discuss both their professional relationship and how they interface with the hospitalist program. They can provide a perspective on the specialist's needs (as it relates to the hospitalist program) as well as the support specialists that provide to the program. They can discuss their level of satisfaction with the program and its impact on their quality of life.

VPMA/CMO

The hospital vice president for medical affairs (VPMA) or chief medical officer (CMO) will discuss the medical staff rules and regulations (e.g., medical staff meeting expectations, committee responsibilities, medical record responsibilities), code of ethics, and quality initiatives. They can also answer any questions related to the medical staff and/or hospital.

Quality Assurance Director

The quality assurance director will discuss the ongoing quality initiatives for both the hospitalist program and the hospital. If the program or hospital has received awards for outstanding performance, this should be shared with the candidate. The director can also discuss hospital information technology initiatives regarding data tracking systems and support programs assisting the hospitalist program achieve its goals.

Hospital Staff

The hospital staff (e.g., nursing director, case managers) will discuss their professional relationship and collaborative efforts with the hospitalist program. They should discuss specific policies, procedures, and programs that have been initiated with the hospitalists to improve patient care and support both hospital staff and hospitalist job satisfaction. They can share their level of satisfaction with the hospitalist program.

Key Community Leaders and Hospital Board Members

The specific participants will depend on the particular circumstances of the candidate. The community leaders and/or board members should connect with the candidate and spouse, providing professional, occupational, and social contacts as appropriate.

Sponsoring Hospital's Medical Staff Coordinator

The medical staff coordinator serves as a resource for the data bank query, licensure status, verification of current clinical privileges, and medical staff status of the physician candidate. They should also confirm medical school graduation, specialty board certification, and run both a criminal background and a credit check.

9.4 DISCUSSION TOPICS

There are many topics to cover during the candidate's site visit. These topics are quite diverse, ranging from school systems to millage rates to hospitalist policies and clinical services offered at the sponsoring hospital. Utilize your recruitment team to discuss this information with the candidate, dividing the work based on subject matter and areas of expertise. The information can be separated into both nonclinical information and clinical information. The following are topics worthy of discussion with the candidate.

Nonclinical Topics

Various nonclinical discussion topics necessitate review with the candidate (and spouse), including community appeal and family, social, and lifestyle factors. These topics can be covered by the recruitment coordinator or hospitalist clinical director. The other hospitalists may also address some of these issues during discussions about the practice opportunity, and the real estate agent will cover many of the topics during the community tour. Exhibit 9.5 outlines essential discussion topics.

Concentrate on topics relevant to the candidate, spouse, and family. If there are topics of particular interest to the candidate (or spouse/family), try to connect him or her with someone of similar interests within your community. Remember, community appeal and lifestyle factors influence recruitment and retention of the candidate *and* spouse/family. Pay attention to all recruitment details, no matter how insignificant they may appear. These details may be vital to the happiness of the spouse/family as well as the candidate. Too many times, recruitment initiatives focus on the employment opportunity at the expense of everything else.

Clinical Topics

A variety of clinical topics warrant discussion with the candidate (refer to Exhibit 9.3 for a detailed list of clinical talking points). These talking points should address information specific to the hospitalist program, sponsoring hospital, and medical community at large (local and outlying). Utilize the hospitalist staff to discuss practice information. Provide information on the operational, administrative, and clinical facets of the practice. Use of supporting materials will be valuable. For example,

Exhibit 9.5 Nonclinical Discussion Topics

Detailed discussion of nonclinical topics is essential to your recruitment efforts. These topics should be discussed with both the candidate and the spouse. The following are examples of discussion topics:

- Community appeal
  - Demography and cultural mix
  - Geography and climate
  - Local economic "health"
    - Availability of affordable housing
    - Cost of living
    - Per capita income
    - Population trends
    - Tax rate/millage rate
    - Major industries and businesses
    - Community services and diversity
  - Neighborhoods (e.g., location, affordability)
  - Safety of the community
  - Neighboring communities
- Family, social, and lifestyle factors
  - Opportunities for spouse
    - Employment/potential work contacts
    - Social (e.g., neighbors, friends, church, civic, community organizations, hobbies)
    - Educational
  - Opportunities for children
    - School system/local colleges
    - Neighborhood and friends
    - Recreational activities (e.g., sporting, arts, natural resources)
  - Cultural events
  - Spiritual resources
  - Dining and entertainment
  - Airport access

share satisfactory survey results, utilization data, and core measure performance to illustrate your points.

Information about the sponsoring hospital and medical community can be provided by the hospital administration, hospital staff, medical staff, and the hospitalists. These persons should address the existing hospital systems that support the clinical, operational, and administrative responsibilities of the medical staff (and hospitalists). Information about the financial health of the hospital can be shared. Specific details about the hospitalist program's relationship with the medical staff, hospital, and hospital administration should also be discussed.

9.5   THE INTERVIEW

You will increase the likelihood of hiring the appropriate physician by developing a coordinated interview process. This requires preparation on the part of your recruitment team. For example, the recruitment team must have a common vision concerning program needs and the type of candidate the practice would like to employ. Developing a list of desired traits the candidate should possess will focus the recruitment team. Prior to the site visit, assemble the team to discuss recruitment goals and each member's roll in the process. Assign specific competencies that each member should explore with the candidate. Allot enough time for each interview so that the candidate can answer questions appropriately without feeling rushed.

Conduct standardized interviews with each candidate. This involves asking each candidate the same set of questions (optimally by the same interviewer) and assessing their responses based on predetermined criteria (see Exhibit 9.6 for a sample interview score card). The questions should be a combination of experience-based (e.g., relating specifically to the candidate's prior work experience), situational-based (e.g., hypothetical situations that may arise on the job), and behavioral descriptive (e.g., inquiring about past performance) questions. This allows all prospective hospitalists to be evaluated in an objective and (potentially) unbiased manner. In some cases you may decide to ask clinical questions or questions based on the unique qualifications that each candidate offers.

During the interview process each interviewer should develop a profile on the candidate. As you interview candidates, pay attention to general appearance, demeanor (including eye contact and speech fluency), general body habitus, and interactive behavior. Particular undesirable behaviors may include late arrival to the interview,

Exhibit 9.6   The Interview Scorecard

The following is a sample scorecard that your recruitment team can use to rank each candidate. There are several categories that may be addressed. The categories address appearance and interpersonal skills, practice compatibility, work ethic, long-term goals and dependability, clinical acumen and experience, and leadership attributes.

Scale:	Unacceptable	Average	Good	Excellent	Need More Information
Appearance	1	2	3	4	×
Interpersonal skills	1	2	3	4	×
Self-confidence	1	2	3	4	×
Values	1	2	3	4	×
Practice fit	1	2	3	4	×
Work ethic	1	2	3	4	×
Adaptability	1	2	3	4	×
Energy level	1	2	3	4	×
Strengths	1	2	3	4	×
Weaknesses	1	2	3	4	×
Long-term goals	1	2	3	4	×
Dependability potential for long-term commitment to area	1	2	3	4	×
Experience as hospitalist	1	2	3	4	×
Clinical knowledge	1	2	3	4	×
Clinical skills	1	2	3	4	×
Judgment	1	2	3	4	×
Leadership skills	1	2	3	4	×
Overall assessment	1	2	3	4	×

Comments:

_____
_____
_____
_____

brusqueness, rudeness, interruptive and/or argumentative speech, inappropriate discussion (e.g., off-color joke, sexual innuendo, slang), and lack of eye contact. Physical characteristics to observe include unkempt appearance, inappropriate attire, restlessness, lack of cleanliness, and disengaged posture.

The observation of desirable characteristics is a start to a candidate's fit into your practice. An engaging, well-groomed candidate with impeccable manners is a good indicator of the candidate's overall interpersonal skills. The observations of promptness, interactive conversation, professional demeanor, and pleasantness further reinforces your decision-making process. It is this particular set of physical characteristics and personal behaviors that will translate into a desirable hire and an ideal representative for your practice. Remember, first impressions are very important. The medical community (e.g., colleagues, hospital staff) and your patients will formulate opinions based on first impressions.

Establish rapport with the candidate early in the interview process. For example, inquire about a hobby, family member, or life experience specific to the candidate. This will demonstrate personal interest in the candidate (rather than interest in the person solely as a hospitalist physician). Make notations during the interview based on factual information (leave interpretations for a later time) and do not pose questions that lead the candidate to a desired response.

Control the interview so that all objectives are met. Pay attention to body language during the interview, as it may provide information about the candidate's feelings. Assess the candidate based on specific criteria created from the job description (e.g., communication skills, leadership skills, judgment). Finally, avoid making conclusions about the candidate until the interview is completed.

Selection of appropriate interview questions will allow the recruitment team to focus on key criteria. Although many of these topics were covered during the telephone screening, they warrant further exploration. During the interview, assess the candidate in general terms. For example, is the candidate well prepared? Does he or she ask intelligent questions? Is the candidate a good communicator? In addition, determine what appeals to the candidate (e.g., high salary, prestigious appointment, technology, autonomy, community, lifestyle). Assessing ambition and whether the candidate is a leader or follower will also be beneficial. To illustrate this point, a highly ambitious physician looking to climb the institutional or professional career ladder may become frustrated working in a small community hospitalist program which offers little room for career advancement. If the candidate is a follower, he or she will need a structured program with effective leadership.

Subsequently, the interview should serve to assess the candidate in a specific manner. This involves queries that assess clinical, analytical, organizational, teaching, and managerial competencies. These qualifications serve to complement any hospitalist program. The depth in exploration of each of these component competencies may vary depending on the position for hire (e.g., clinical director, academic position, quality assurance director). This evaluation involves the method of structured interviewing, which utilizes behavioral descriptive interview techniques.

Structured Interview Questions

The structured approach in an interview utilizes competency-based (sometimes called evidence- or experience-based) interview questions. The objective of this approach is to standardize the process and make it as unbiased as possible. This line of questioning targets the core competencies of the physician and focuses on the candidate's prior work experience. You should follow up this inquiry with in-depth, probing questions to ensure that the person possesses the necessary skills to perform effectively. To accomplish the desired results, you may choose to ask direct questions, such as:

- How would you rate your skills in the intensive care unit?
- How would you rate your procedural skills?
- How would you rate your communication skills?
- How would you rate your ability to treat chronically ill patients?
- Describe your leadership philosophy.
- In what ways are you a team player?
- How would your current clinical director rate your time management skills?
- How would you rate your administrative skills?
- How would you rate your business skills as it relates to medicine?

Questions such as *"What is the level of your diagnostic skills compared to your bedside manner?"* or *"Would you rather admit a patient with acute respiratory distress or one with multiple psycho-social issues?"* are structured questions that require a candidate to compare skills sets or preferences and are used to uncover an applicant's weaknesses. The structured line of questioning allows you to accomplish several things. First, it provides insight into the candidate's skills and lets you compare and contrast them with your program's needs. In addition, the candidate may reveal his or her philosophy on a given subject. This information will assist you as you assess for common vision and values (between the practice and the candidate). Finally, this line of questioning allows the candidate to demonstrate his or her analytical skills. For example, your program may be experiencing a problem with coding and chart documentation which is affecting reimbursement from payors (and thus, your bottom line). By asking the candidate to rate his or her business skills relating to the practice of medicine, you can assess coding experience and knowledge of chart documentation requirements. You may also gain insight into the candidate's philosophy on the integration of business and medicine in today's world.

The following example illustrates the line of questioning you may pursue to evaluate the candidate's business skills. It opens with a structured question and follows up with probing inquiries. The candidate discusses his or her skills and reveals additional (philosophical) information concerning the current payor system in the United States.

Interviewer: How would you rate your business skills as they relate to medicine?

Candidate: I think they're good. I'm certainly aware of the need to practice cost-effective medicine, especially with pay-for-performance programs ... and we all know the troubles associated with Medicare.

Interviewer: Can you tell me how you address this problem with Medicare in your current program?

Candidate: We have an excellent practice manager who provides assistance so we can capture all of our charges. We have monthly meetings and discuss how we can do a better job.

Interviewer: Who performs the coding in your practice?

Candidate: In the past we had a coding specialist who did this work, but in the last year, because of cutbacks, we are expected to do our own coding.

Interviewer: Do you feel comfortable coding, and is your performance evaluated?

Candidate: Now I feel comfortable but I didn't when we first started to code our own charts. I have to thank our practice manager, who provided coding reviews and feedback until we got it right. Currently, we are evaluated each month by having 10 charts audited for chart documentation and coding accuracy. We get feedback about our performance at our monthly meeting, which is very helpful. As doctors we were never trained in business, but it's becoming especially important to learn on the job. It's only going to get worse in the future with Medicare cutbacks and the uncertainties that face our profession. Everyone talks about universal healthcare but where's the money going to come from?

Interviewer: What do you think we have to do to prepare ourselves for the future?

Candidate: I think we need to work together to build a system in which we maximize efficiencies and drive the costs of medicine down while not compromising patient care. The patient comes first; that is why I got into medicine in the first place....

Situational Questions

Situational or behavioral descriptive questioning focuses on how the candidate performed in past circumstances. Situational questions explore the physician's problem-solving approach, eliciting information about analytical skills. It also provides information on how the person may perform under pressure and/or unexpected circumstances. Thinking on one's feet is critical for effective hospitalist performance.

A behavioral line of questioning allows the physician to share his or her experiences of past performance. This line of questioning reasons that past behavior may help predict future performance. Behavioral questioning asks the candidate "*What did you do?*" in a past situation, or "*Tell me about a time when you ...?*" while situational questioning asks "*What would you do?*" or "*What if ?.*" Behavioral interviewing techniques utilize open-ended questions. In some situations, the answers are compared to a list of previously determined acceptable answers (in an attempt to objectify the process). The following are examples of behavioral questions:

- How do you deal with drug-abusing patients?
- Tell me about a time when you demonstrated excellent leadership skills.
- Tell me how you interact with referring physicians who you believe are incompetent.
- How do you deal with patients in need of outpatient follow-up who do not want to return to their current PCP?
- What do you do when you have a colleague who is dumping his or her work on you?
- Describe a situation where you had to had to tell a patient that he or she had cancer.

- Tell me how you resolved a difficult situation with a colleague.
- Tell me about a situation in which you took charge that led to positive results.

Once you have received an answer, don't be afraid to explore further. For example, you may ask the candidate *"How did you do that?"* or *"Tell me exactly what steps you took to resolve that problem?"* or *"On what did you base your decision?"*

Consider the following scenario: Your program has been experiencing significant problems with customer service. PCPs, patients, and nursing staff (at the sponsoring hospital) are disenfranchised with the program. Performance on the satisfaction surveys is below expectations and the PCPs are threatening to refer their patients to the competing hospitalist program in the community (who admit to another hospital). This will obviously create problems for your program and may jeopardize the subsidy provided by the sponsoring hospital. Your program's clinical director, who was a part of the problem, has recently departed and you're currently recruiting for a replacement. The recruitment team resolves to focus recruitment of a hospitalist who possesses both excellent customer service and leadership skills. The following will illustrate the application of behavioral questioning to obtain the information you would like to evaluate.

Interviewer: Tell me how you resolved a difficult situation with a colleague.

Candidate: One time when we were understaffed I helped solve the staffing situation until we became fully staffed. We had a doctor who refused to pull his share of the load.

Interviewer: Tell me exactly what steps you took to resolve the problem.

Candidate: First, I asked the doctor why he was resistant to help the practice and his colleagues during this difficult time. The doctor had young children and told me he didn't want to be away from his family more than he already was. I asked him what time of day was more important for him to be home. He wanted to be home for dinner because his two sons were at daycare all day and they went to bed by 7:30 p.m. So I told him I would cover those times in his additional shifts if he would agree to work more until we hired another doctor. He agreed and things worked out for all of us.

Interviewer: Why did you do that?

Candidate: There were several reasons. First, someone had to see the patient—that's what we get paid to do. Second, having the doctor work part of the shift was better than having him work none at all. It met his needs and it met our needs as a practice. Third, that was the right thing to do for our patients and hospitalist program....

Situational questions are those that pose hypothetical examples in order to evaluate a candidate's ability to think critically and logically. These questions require the physician to problem solve. Look for responses that are relevant and consistent. Listen carefully to how the candidate analyzed and managed the specific problem. Examples of this line of questioning:

- If you were asked to admit a patient by a PCP who is very supportive of your program and you didn't feel hospitalization was appropriate, how would you deal with that?
- If you were the only hospitalist on call at night and you had five critically ill patients to admit at the same time, how would you deal with that?
- If the administrator of your hospital, from whom you receive subsidy, asked you to admit more patients to the hospital because the census was low, what would you do?
- If you assume care of a patient who you believe received substandard or even incompetent care, what would you do?
- What would you do if a specialist refused to come into the hospital in the middle of the night to see a patient who was unstable and rapidly declining?

The following line of questioning illustrates this approach.

Interviewer: If you were the only hospitalist on call at night and you had five critically ill patients to admit at the same time, how would you deal with this problem?

Candidate: I would assess who the sickest patients were and decide what I needed to do to get them stabilized.

Interviewer: What if they all were equally unstable and in need of immediate care?

Candidate: I would do several things. I would see if the emergency department physicians could assist me. I would also ask for help from the intensive care and emergency department nursing staff. Finally, I would call my hospitalist partners if I got desperate.

Interviewer: Why did you specifically mention the intensive care nurses?

Candidate: For two reasons. First, they are trained to deal with critically ill patients, and second, that's where these patients would ultimately be transferred....

Indirect Questions

Indirect questioning solicits broad responses from a candidate. It allows the candidate an opportunity to direct the conversation. Additionally, it provides the interviewer with insight into both the candidate's thought process and the ability to organize and formulate his or her thoughts. Indirect questions may also elicit personal information about the physician, depending on the candidate's focus. It is always interesting to see how a candidate handles an open line of questioning. Examples of nondirect questions:

- Tell me about yourself
- Tell me about your experience
- How did you get to where you are today?
- What are your professional expectations?
- Discuss the role of the hospitalist today
- Can you tell me more about that?
- What do you think about the future of medicine?
- Tell me about your last job
- How would you evaluate your present practice?

You may follow up this line of questioning with more directed or situational questions. This will provide insight into the mind of the physician while also obtaining objective information. It will also allow you to evaluate the candidate's thought processes in terms of consistency and reliability. An example of this line of questioning:

Interviewer: How did you get to where you are today?

Candidate: My father was a doctor and I really admired him. He helped so many people in his lifetime and I wanted to follow in his shoes.

Interviewer: What kind of doctor was he?

Candidate: He was a hematologist.

Interviewer: Why didn't you specialize in hematology if you wanted to follow in his footsteps?

Candidate: Well, I wasn't sure what field of medicine I wanted to go into until my third year of residency. Hematology was always a consideration, but I thought I could help more patients if I went into hospitalist medicine.

Interviewer: What other influences helped you to be the person you are today?

Candidate: My mother. She always showed kindness and empathy to everyone and I think it rubbed off on me. She was certainly a big influence on me growing up and on me as an adult. Some of my attending physicians in residency influenced me as well.

Interviewer: How did they influence you?

Candidate: Dr. Jones taught me how to let a patient die with dignity. We're trained as doctors to preserve life at all costs, but he showed me how we could be good doctors yet be able to let go.

Interviewer: Do you have experience with palliative care teams, and if so, how?

Candidate: Yes, I actually did a one-month rotation with a palliative care team. I learned a lot about chronic diseases and appropriate resource utilization....

In the example above, the interviewer was able to obtain information about the candidate's role models and family background, philosophy, professional values, and interpersonal skills.

Direct Questions

There are many direct questions that you can ask a candidate during the interview process. The format is simple and it allows you to gather a great deal of clinical, personal, ethical, and philosophical information about the candidate. These questions may provide insight into the candidate's future goals and aspirations. They may elicit responses regarding the physician's business acumen. In addition, you can obtain information regarding candidate and spousal expectations, their familiarity with life (climate, culture, recreational, etc.) in a similar community, and whether or not they have family living in close proximity. Exhibit 9.7 provides a list of sample questions.

Exhibit 9.7   Direct Interview Questions

Depending on the choice of questions, you can gather information about the physician and spouse regarding a number of topics. The following are examples of direct questions.

- Discuss your philosophy on communication with the PCP.
- Discuss your previous experiences with hospital administrators.
- What skills do you have that relate to this position?
- What were your responsibilities in the XYZ hospitalist program?
- How many patients a day did you see?
- What is your greatest strength?
- What is your greatest weakness?
- What motivates you?
- How do you define success?
- What do you think it takes to be a successful hospitalist?
- Of what personal accomplishments are you most proud?
- If you were to credit one person for being responsible for your success, who would that be?
- What are your long-term plans?
- Why are you looking for new employment?
- What are the primary factors that you and your spouse are seeking in a new location?
- Have you or your spouse lived in this part of the country previously?
- Have you or your spouse previously resided in a community of this size?
- Why do you want to work here?
- What has been your biggest professional challenge?
- What has been your biggest personal challenge?
- What do you see as the greatest challenge facing hospitalists today? In the future?
- What do you feel you can offer our program?
- Why should we hire you?
- What other practice opportunities are you considering?
- How would you describe the ideal job?
- Why did you choose to be a hospitalist?
- What goals do you have in your career?

- How do you handle stress?
- How do you deal with conflict?
- How do you deal with success?
- What are five traits of successful hospitalists?
- What should the priorities of a hospitalist clinical director be?
- Discuss your experience relating to physician performance analysis (e.g., clinical and financial).
- What should the priorities of a hospitalist be?
- What do you do for fun?

Illegal Interview Questions

Knowing what questions you can't ask a candidate is very important in the recruitment process. There are various federal, state, and local laws regulating the questions that a prospective employer can ask a candidate. There are several topics you must broach with caution. You should not ask about race, religion, color, national origin, birthplace, gender, age, disability, or marital/family status because if you base your hiring decision on any of these answers, it is discriminatory. The following are examples of subjects you should be careful approaching:

- *Immigration status.* If you're interested in immigration status for legal/visa purposes, you cannot ask *"Are you a U.S. citizen?"* or *"Where were you born?"* You can ask *"Are you authorized to work in the United States?"*
- *Affiliations.* If you're interested in the physician's professional affiliations that may affect your practice in a positive manner, you cannot ask *"What local or national medical societies do you belong to?"* You can ask *"Do you belong to any professional associations that you consider relevant to performing this job?"*
- *Marital and/or family status.* If you're uncertain about whether a candidate will be willing to relocate to your community because of spousal influence, you cannot ask *"Are you married?"* or *"Who do you live with?"* You can ask *"Is there anything that will prevent you from relocating into this community?"*
- *Disabilities.* If you are concerned whether the candidate can perform the essential functions of the job, you cannot ask *"Do you have any disabilities?"* or *"What was the date of your last complete physical exam?"* You can ask *"Are you able to perform*

the essential functions of this job with or without reasonable accommodation?"

- *Criminal record.* If you are concerned about any legal difficulties that a candidate may have that would limit his or her ability to obtain a medical license or practice medicine, you cannot ask *"Have you ever been arrested?"* You can ask *"Have you ever been convicted of …?"*

- *Military.* Losing a physician to military duty can be very disruptive to your program. If you're interested in learning about a candidate's commitment, you cannot ask *"Are you a member of the national guard?"* You can ask *"Do you have any upcoming activities that would require extensive time away from the practice?"*

- *Religion.* Some candidates may have religious beliefs that might limit their availability to work. You can't ask *"Which religious holidays do you observe?"* You can ask *"Are you able to work within our required schedule?"*

Hiring the ideal candidate for your program is very challenging and a multifactorial feat. Selection of appropriate interview questions and avoidance of illegal questions will facilitate the recruitment process. The information gleaned from these questions will provide your recruitment team with an objective basis with which to make a decision. However, some experts believe that the traditional interview process is flawed, as every human being is influenced by first impressions, personal beliefs, and other biases that affect both the interview process and employee selection. Kevin C. Wooten (associate professor of management and human resources at the University of Houston–Clear Lake) postulates that in the future recruitment may utilize Web-based technologies (such as videoconferencing) and personality testing (along with the more traditional approaches) to neutralize this potential bias. In the end the recruitment process must still rely on the face-to-face exchange between potential employee and employer. Meticulous preparation and flawless execution of the recruitment plan will minimize the risk of selection bias.

9.6   THE POSTVISIT PHASE

Provide the candidate with a copy of the contract template at the conclusion of the site visit and prior to his or her departure. This gives the candidate an idea of the contract parameters if an offer is made (contract specifics are discussed in Chapter 10). If the candidate is exceptional, an official offer can be made prior to departure. In most instances the salary is left blank on the contract until the recruitment team can be queried about the candidate.

Require all participants in the recruitment process to provide feedback on the candidate within 24 to 48 hours of the site visit. People performing interviews should complete an evaluation of the candidate within this same time frame (see Exhibit 9.6). Set up a teleconference or meeting between the recruitment team leaders, optimally within 72 hours of the site visit. These leaders may include the hospitalist administrator, hospitalist clinical director, and the hospital CEO or COO (if the program is hospital owned) to discuss whether an offer will be made and, if affirmative, at what salary and signing perks.

If your program is extending an offer, the clinical director should contact the candidate within 72 hours of the site visit, answering any questions and communicating the program's interest in the candidate. Solicit any outstanding references during this time frame. Send the candidate a formal letter as well (by e-mail, fax, or mail) with an official job offer and contract. In the event that your program has additional candidates for the position, extend your offer with a timeline for acceptance so you don't risk losing these other physicians. If you're not extending an offer, send a letter thanking the candidate for his or her interest. Also, if a recruitment agency is involved, inform them about your decision.

9.7   HIRING PROTOCOL

Send an application packet to the candidate with the official job offer and contract. This packet should include the following:

- State medical license application
- Drug enforcement agency (DEA) certificate application
- Hospital medical staff application
- Credentialing package for insurance carriers
- Professional liability insurance application
- Benefits package

Have the candidate schedule an appointment with the human resource department within your practice or it can be outsourced to the hospital or another company. This department should arrange for health screening of the employee and for a preemployment physical examination. Human resources must also review the benefit package with the new physician and provide assistance if needed regarding selection of benefits. The practice manager should monitor this process and ensure that it proceeds expeditiously. The goal is to have all applications and materials completed by the new hospitalist and returned to the practice manager within 10 to 14 days of job acceptance.

10 The Contract

An effective physician employment agreement or contract defines the essential responsibilities and obligations of both the employee and the employer. Specifically, it addresses the terms of engagement between the physician and employer, including the employment arrangement, qualifications, standards of service, physician services, duties and responsibilities of the employer, and the term of employment. It defines the financial parameters of the contract, such as hours of employment, compensation (e.g., salary and/or incentive), benefits, professional liability, and employment activities outside the practice. The contract also addresses legal provisions including restrictive covenants, termination of employment, patient record ownership, confidentiality, and the financial relationship between employer and physician. The content of the contract will vary depending on both the contractual arrangement and the employer (e.g., private practice vs. hospital employed vs. management company). This chapter serves only as a guide and is not meant to provide legal advice. The contract should be written by legal counsel specializing in healthcare.

10.1 EMPLOYMENT ARRANGEMENT

The employment arrangement defines the specific professional relationship between the involved parties. For example, it defines the employer (e.g., parent company or subsidiary), employee, and the physician's title (e.g., hospitalist).

10.2 QUALIFICATIONS

This section of the contract describes the conditions of employment for the physician. These are conditions that must be fulfilled in order for

Hospitalist Recruitment and Retention: Building a Hospital Medicine Program,
By Kenneth G. Simone
Copyright © 2010 Wiley-Blackwell

the doctor to perform his or her job responsibilities. For example, it should state that the physician must:

- Maintain a valid and unrestricted license to practice medicine in the particular state or states of employment
- Be an active member of the medical staff (at the sponsoring hospital) with full privileges and in good standing
- Possess a valid DEA number with full licensure to prescribe all medications, including narcotics
- Be a participating provider in third-party insurance programs such as Medicare and Medicaid
- Be a member in various health maintenance organizations (HMOs), preferred provider organizations (PPOs), and other organizations deemed essential by the employer
- Maintain eligibility and remain insured under the professional liability insurance coverage of the practice
- Become or maintain board certification in his or her specialty field

10.3 STANDARDS OF SERVICE

The standards of service section typically outlines practice standards under which the physician is held accountable. The intent of this section is twofold; it serves as a guide for the physician and it protects the employer in the event that there's significant deviation in the medical care provided by this person. The content may include a clause stipulating that the physician must retain independent judgment and responsibility in the practice of hospitalist medicine and perform his or her duties in accordance with:

- The practice procedures created to ensure high-quality medical care
- All applicable federal and state statutes and regulations
- The currently acceptable and approved methods and practices applicable to the relevant specialty board
- The requirements of the state medical licensure board
- The standards and recommendations of the Joint Commission
- The mission, objectives, policies, and procedures of both the practice and sponsoring hospital (including medical staff bylaws and hospital regulations)

10.4   PHYSICIAN SERVICES

The practice must describe the duties and responsibilities of the employed physician (e.g., "physician services") in the contract. This section defines the day-to-day hospitalist tasks such as managing all aspects of a patient's care, coordinating care with the referring physician/PCP, supervising support staff (if applicable), performing record-keeping activities, and participating in administrative duties. The contract should also state that the physician will abide by all of the rules, regulations, and responsibilities that come with active membership on the sponsoring hospital's medical staff.

10.5   DUTIES AND RESPONSIBILITIES OF THE EMPLOYER

The employer should define the services provided to the practice (and their employed physicians). The employer typically provides practice management services, billing and collection services, expertise regarding regulatory compliance [e.g., Health Insurance Portability and Accountability Act (HIPAA), Occupational Safety and Health Administration (OSHA)], support staff (with supervision), office space, supplies, and equipment.

10.6   THE TERM OF EMPLOYMENT

The term of employment delineates the length of the contact. Most contracts are written for one to three years. It may be an evergreen contract, implying that the terms of the agreement will be extended automatically for another year unless either party notifies the other in writing. It is prudent to specify how much notice is required by either party wishing to terminate the contract *at any time* during the contract. Most agreements call for 90 to 180 days' notice.

In the event that your program employs an IMG, verbiage should be written emphasizing that the physician must adhere to the U.S. immigration laws. The contract should protect the program from any physician failing to meet the conditions of his or her admission to the United States. It should also protect the program from any physician not authorized to work in the United States or within your program.

10.7   HOURS OF EMPLOYMENT

Some programs address physician workload in the contract. Workload may be defined by the number of hours per day, week, or year, or by the number of days or shifts per week or year. Additionally, programs may specify the number of call nights, weekends, and holidays that the physician is required to work each year. Defining the *specific* workload is not advised, as they are many variables that can affect this. However, it is reasonable to provide the current practice model in an attached schedule (e.g., one week on–one week off model, rotating call model with five-day workweek and every fourth night and fourth weekend on call) with the caveat that the practice retains the final decision-making authority regarding changes to the schedule. This will provide the physician with a general idea of the expected workload while allowing the practice flexibility in the event of unexpected occurrences (e.g., staffing shortage, high census).

10.8 COMPENSATION

The compensation portion of the contract addresses the physician's annual salary, payment schedule (e.g., weekly, biweekly) and benefits. The benefit package may include CME (monetary allowance), health and dental insurance (physician only or physician and family), life insurance, disability insurance, malpractice insurance, retirement plan (with or without a profit-sharing match), professional amenities (e.g., books, journal subscriptions, license fees, cell phone and other equipment), moving expenses, sign-on bonus, and medical school loan repayment. In the event that your program has an incentive or bonus plan, the payment schedule should be defined (e.g., monthly, quarterly). The incentive plan specifics should be described in a separate document, as plans are subject to change annually (e.g., focus, metrics, percent bonus money allotted per target). Finally, the practice should define the amount of time allotted for vacation, CME, maternity/paternity leave, sick leave, and sabbatical, if applicable.

10.9 PROFESSIONAL LIABILITY

Many programs require the physician to pay a portion of the tail coverage (protection for liability claims made in the future) if he or she leaves the practice prior to completion of the employment agreement. Usually, it is allocated according to the number of years the physician is employed by the practice:

- 0–11 months employed: physician assumes 100% of the premium tail
- 12–23 months employed: physician assumes 67% of the premium tail
- 24–35 months employed: physician assumes 33% of the premium tail
- 36 months employed: practice assumes 100% of the premium tail

10.10   EMPLOYMENT ACTIVITIES OUTSIDE THE PRACTICE

Some practices forbid the employed physician from working in another capacity while under contract to the hospitalist program (e.g., moonlighting, specialty clinics). If this is the case with your program, it is prudent to state this in the employment contract. For example, it may be stated that the physician shall devote all of his or her professional time to the practice. Alternatively, it may state that the physician is not allowed to participate in activities deemed competitive or adverse to the practice (e.g., less restrictive). The practice should critically evaluate whether it will place restrictions on the physician, as this may be deleterious to recruitment.

10.11   RESTRICTIVE COVENANTS

Depending on the employment arrangement and state law, the contract may include a restrictive covenant (or noncompete clause) prohibiting the physician from working for a hospitalist program felt to be in direct competition with the employer. Stark III has eased regulations for practices receiving recruitment assistance from a hospital by allowing the practice to impose a reasonable restrictive covenant to recruit a physician new to the area [15]. The noncompete clause must be reasonable in both geographic distance (from the current practice) and length of time (before the physician can return to the local community and work for a competitor). Discuss what's considered legally "reasonable" in your community with your attorney. The clause may also include a buy-out which allows the physician to pay a reasonable fee to the practice for the freedom to practice without restriction.

The use of a restrictive covenant in hospitalist medicine is controversial in that the hospitalist practice does not have a patient panel but, rather, treats patients referred from other physicians or hospitals. Thus, opponents of restrictive covenants contend that a hospitalist cannot take patients with them if they leave a practice. Although this is true, hospitalists can influence to which hospitalist practice and/or hospital referring providers send their patients.

10.12 TERMINATION OF EMPLOYMENT

In this section the process for contract termination by either the practice or the physician is defined. Typically, a professional relationship such as this requires at least a 90-day notice on either party's part to terminate the contract without cause. Notice should be provided in writing and by certified mail (with a return receipt requested). This section should also define conditions under which the physician can be terminated with cause. The following are examples of such conditions:

- Physician is unable to carry out his or her employment responsibilities for 90 days out of a 180-day period
- Physician fails to maintain the "Qualifications" or "Standards of Service" defined in the contract
- Physician's license is either revoked by the state medical association or substantially limits his or her ability to practice medicine and fulfill the obligations designated under "Physician Services"
- Physician commits a crime or participates in criminal misconduct, significantly reducing his or her effectiveness in performing his or her employment responsibilities
- Physician participates in activities that have a negative impact on the operations and/or reputation of the practice
- Physician is providing inadequate patient care and/or placing the patients' well-being at risk
- Physician fails to abide by the terms of the contract and/or provide all of the services defined in the employment agreement (under "Physician Services")
- Physician fails to maintain immigration status or the physician's immigration status changes, rendering him or her unlawfully present or unauthorized to work legally in the United States (or the physician cannot reenter the states)

The contract should state that the practice has no further obligations if the physician is terminated for cause (unless physician compensation for services provided *prior to* the termination is outstanding). The practice may provide a clause describing conditions under which the physician may terminate the contract with cause, such as the practice's failure to comply with the financial obligations of the contract.

10.13 PATIENT RECORD OWNERSHIP

Many programs maintain patient records (e.g., admission history and physical reports, consultations, labs, diagnostic studies, discharge summaries) on all patients cared for by the practice. Therefore, it should be stated in the contract that all patient records and files relating to inpatients cared for by the hospitalist physicians remain the property of the practice. This will prohibit a physician who is leaving the practice from taking patient records with him or her.

10.14 CONFIDENTIALITY

Maintenance of patient confidentiality should be a major focus for all physicians and practices. This section should clearly state that strict confidentiality must be maintained at all times and that the physician must abide by HIPAA regulations. If your program is in a highly competitive area (e.g., with multiple hospitalist programs), consider adding a confidentiality clause prohibiting the physician from sharing proprietary information about the program (including financial, operational, or strategic information).

10.15 FINANCIAL RELATIONSHIP BETWEEN EMPLOYER AND PHYSICIAN

This clause requires the physician to disclose any ownership, investment, or compensation arrangement that he or she (or the family) may have with any entity providing health services. It should also state that the physician's compensation is based solely on the services contracted (e.g., the physician receives no subsidy for referrals or services ordered at the sponsoring hospital). This section must be present in the contract to comply with Stark I and Stark II regulations.

In summary, create an employment contract that is fair to both parties. The agreement should define the expectations and obligations of both physician and employer. The terms of the agreement and compensation should be clear. Be thorough in your approach, yet keep it simple. Consult with your healthcare legal counsel and remember: Effective and defensible contracts protect the rights of the employer as well as those of the employee.

11 Practice Management Strategies

Now that your program has a recruitment and retention plan in place, its implementation will be very challenging. Many programs develop elaborate plans but fail in the implementation phase. Successful launch requires both effective leadership and management of the practice. Development of operational policies will guide both the process and your program to succeed. In this chapter we discuss practice management strategies allowing your program to attract exceptional hospitalist candidates *and* retain them. We provide recommendations for practice infrastructure. It will also allow for the systematic determination of staffing needs. When your hospitalist program has an effective management plan in place allowing its physicians to thrive, it will support both retention and ultimately, program success.

Appropriate staffing numbers and team composition will help support recruitment, retention, and practice stability. Staff stability provides for the delivery of quality care and ultimately, patient satisfaction. It also supports job satisfaction for both hospitalist provider and hospital staff. An appropriately staffed practice improves the likelihood of provider efficiency and cost-effectiveness. A fully staffed practice allows your program to offer comprehensive services to the hospital and community.

Many elements are involved in an effective practice management plan. Only those components that affect recruitment and retention are covered in this chapter.

11.1 THE HOSPITALIST BUDGET

Your program's budget will be a guiding factor for the number and composition of clinical staff as well as the practice model (discussed in Chapter 5) and scope of services offered by the program. For example,

Hospitalist Recruitment and Retention: Building a Hospital Medicine Program,
By Kenneth G. Simone
Copyright © 2010 Wiley-Blackwell

if the program has $1 million budgeted for providers, you must decide how to distribute these funds. As part of this process you will estimate the number of providers required to run the practice effectively. This includes consideration of the cost for a particular provider (e.g., physician vs. NPC, subspecialist vs. internist or family practitioner) as well as the ability of the provider to cover his or her costs. For example, an NPC is approximately two-thirds the cost of a pediatric hospitalist and one-half the cost of an adult hospitalist [9]. NPCs must be supervised by a physician (in a hospital setting). In addition, NPCs are limited in their clinical abilities (compared to physicians), and potentially, in their ability to generate revenue. Therefore, your program must balance the cost savings of hiring an NPC with their limitations. This must be superimposed over other considerations, such as your program's scope of service. There are many other factors that guide the determination of both staff size and composition, and they are discussed in detail in Section 11.2.

The budget process will vary depending on employment model (e.g., hospital owned, local hospitalist only, management company). The hospital-owned model is addressed in this chapter to illustrate the need for collaboration. In this model the hospital subsidizes the program to provide specific services, which may include, but not be limited to, direct patient care, committee work, medical staff and hospital leadership, teaching, and emergency department call coverage. In return for this support the hospital may have several expectations (see Exhibit 11.1). Once all involved parties are aware of the responsibilities and expectations, productive discussion can occur regarding the annual budget.

The budget process should be consistent from year to year, including the review period (e.g., beginning or midway into the fourth quarter), the participants (e.g., hospitalist administrator, hospital chief financial officer, hospitalist clinical director, hospitalist practice manager), and the data evaluated (see Exhibit 11.2). Allow ample time to review the data prior to meeting. Encourage the clinical director's active participation in the budget process. If the hospitalist providers believe that they have a voice in the budgeting process, they will buy into the final budget. Physician input is also important for another reason; the providers work in the trenches and have firsthand understanding of program requirements.

11.2   HOSPITALIST STAFFING

Determination of staff composition and staff size may be derived in several ways. Your program budget will play a significant role in this

Exhibit 11.1   Hospital Expectations

Every hospital should anticipate a positive return on investment from the hospitalist practice—if not in the immediate short term, than certainly in the long term. The hospitalist program may be expected to:

- Provide cost savings for the hospital (e.g., through responsible resource management and decreased length of stay, the 30-day readmission rate, the cost per case).
- Improve the quality of patient care (e.g., hospitalist development of evidence-based patient care guidelines and innovative care systems).
- Provide community service (e.g., hospital care for indigent patients).
- Support the medical staff in the community (e.g., providing inpatient care for PCP and specialist patients, offering surgical co-management services, covering the code blue and rapid-response teams).

Exhibit 11.2   Budgetary Data

There are a number of metrics that your program may analyze through the budget process. The specific metrics will depend on the hospital's ability to access the data and to ensure that they are accurate, comprehensive, timely, and reproducible. The following information will be valuable in the budget process:

- Program utilization (e.g., ADC, number of admissions/discharges, number of consultations, annual billable encounters)
- Billing data (e.g., gross charges and net receipts, collection ratios, payor mix, top 10 DRGs, referral sources)
- Financial performance: provider and practice (e.g., RVUs, coding and chart documentation, ALOS, average cost per case, ancillary utilization)
- Clinical performance: provider and practice (e.g., 30-day readmission rate, complication rate, mortality rate, core measure performance, patient satisfaction, PCP satisfaction)

Exhibit 11.3   Factors Influencing Hospitalist Staffing

Several factors are worth consideration in the determination of staff size and composition. Some or all of these factors may influence your program's staffing. These include:

- Program utilization
- Patient acuity
- Program scope of service
- Provider availability
- Provider contract hours per year
- Practice culture
- Community standards
- Geographic location

process as noted in Section 11.1. There are several other factors that influence staffing (see Exhibit 11.3). Some or all of these factors may provide a challenge to your program. Patient acuity and program scope of service are two of the more common considerations.

Program Utilization and Patient Acuity

Program utilization is a large driver of hospitalist staffing. *Utilization* refers to the ADC of the program, the number of admissions and consultations per year, and the number of encounters per year. These metrics provide a rough idea of the workload intensity. An accurate assessment can only be made after considering other factors, including the acuity level of these patients as well as the added-value services (not measured by the metrics above) provided by the hospitalists. Once this is established, an estimate can be made regarding the number of clinical hours required to cover the program each year. This in turn will drive the program's staffing needs.

The following real-life example will illustrate this point. Program X has an average daily census of 38 patients. In addition to direct patient care responsibilities, the providers participate in code blue and rapid-response team coverage, serve on key hospital committees, and provide preoperative medical clearance for patients admitted though the emergency department for emergency surgery (e.g., hip fracture, acute abdomen). The program employs eight physicians and four NPCs.

These providers work in a seven on/seven off schedule and are hospital employed. During the annual budget process the hospitalist clinical director requested a ninth physician and was given the OK (without resistance from hospital administration).

Focusing on the ADC, it may appear that the program is overstaffed (e.g., four physicians and two NPCs work each day), as the ADC would be less than 10 patients per physician. When you consider that one of the physicians (along with the NPCs) is utilized in nonclinical duties *each* day (at approximately one-half of an FTE) and one physician is assigned to the night shift (in-house), it becomes clear that this is not the case. Hospital administration found value in the program's scope of service (e.g., they looked beyond ADC per physician) and subsidized the additional physician without opposition. Administration is especially pleased because the number of surgeries (and surgeon satisfaction) has increased in the hospital in the past year (there is a competing hospital within the community). They are also gratified to note resolution of the emergency department code blue coverage problem. Resolution of these problems was attributed to the hospitalist program's assistance with preoperative consultations and 24/7 code blue coverage.

Program Scope of Service

The program's scope of service refers to all activities and responsibilities performed by hospitalists within the practice. These activities may include direct patient contact, such as medical management of hospitalized patients, consultative work, procedural work, palliative care services, and perioperative services. Hospitalist duties may include call coverage such as emergency department on-call coverage and code blue and rapid-response team coverage. Finally, they may also include administrative, supervisory, and educational duties such as medical staff committee work, medical staff leadership appointments, management of an observation or LTAC unit, and teaching responsibilities (e.g., medical students, interns, residents, hospital staff). It is a challenge trying to quantify both the amount of work performed and the time required by a provider to accomplish these activities as well as the number of providers needed to accomplish the program's tasks. Not all of these activities are reimbursable by insurers; thus, additional subsidy may be required from another source (e.g., the sponsoring hospital).

Some of the hospitalist's activities cannot be quantified for staffing purposes by the metrics listed in Exhibit 11.2. Thus, staffing estimates must take into consideration the time required to provide these services. For example, if your program provides around-the-clock code blue and rapid-response team coverage, this service should be quantified by the number of provider hours required to provide this service. Program scope of service may also influence the composition of your staff. Some activities do not require direct physician involvement, and NPCs may represent a more cost-effective means of delivering these services.

Provider Availability, Geographic Location, and Community Standards

The composition of your clinical staff may be affected by a number of nonfinancial factors. When recruiting, your choice of candidate will be directly related to the availability of physicians in a specific specialty as well as the candidate pool (e.g., those wishing to submit a CV for consideration). The applicant pool will be influenced by the mode(s) of advertising chosen to identify (and attract) candidates (see Chapter 4). It will also be influenced by the specific information provided in the job posting. For example, the posting may identify a specific specialty (e.g., internist, FP, IM–pediatrics), may designate board eligibility/certification requirements, and may specify preferred experience level and skill sets. Thus, your program's decisions about the optimal candidate directly affect the recruitment search as well as how inclusive or exclusive the search should be.

Community standards may also play a role in your candidate search. For example, if your hospital has a closed ICU, an intensivist may be required to provide care for the program's ICU patients. Also, if your program is considering employment of a NPC, review the sponsoring hospital's medical staff bylaws prior to making a decision. Utilization of NPCs will be guided by the bylaws at your hospital. The amount of autonomy allowed NPCs will vary depending on the institution, which may make hiring of these providers more or less attractive to your program. Additionally, if your referral base has significant concerns about NPCs treating their patients (and there are competing hospitalist programs in the community), it could affect your market share.

Provider choice may also be influenced by the geographic location of your program. For example, if your program is located in a rural area, an IMG candidate may be ideal, based on his or her visa status (see Chapter 1). A FP or IM–pediatric hospitalist would be reasonable specialty choices as well, as they provide great flexibility in the care of adult and pediatric patients. Finally, NPCs may also be a good choice, based on the cost to your program and clinical versatility.

NPC Utilization

A book on hospitalist recruitment and retention would be remiss without discussing the utilization of NPCs within your practice. If your program plans to hire a NPC, ensure the buy-in of all physicians within your practice. It is important to define the NPC's role and expectations prior to the start date (see Exhibit 11.4). Educate both the hospitalist and hospital staff early in the process, creating awareness about the NPC's role. If there is confusion or resistance (even from one physician), it can undermine the NPC as well as your program. It may also affect how the NPC is utilized when the dissenting physician is working.

Exhibit 11.4   NPC Responsibilities

The NPC's role and expectations vary according to the hospitalist program. This is a consequence of program philosophy, community standards, and state regulations. Common responsibilities of NPCs may include the following:

- Provides direct patient care (typically, rounding on less acute patients)
- Screens admissions in the emergency department
- Provides history and physical examinations on all patients admitted to the program
- Participates in the discharge of all patients (e.g., coordinates with discharge planners/case managers, writes prescriptions, provides patient and family education, arranges for outpatient follow-up with PCP, coordinates the scheduling of outpatient studies, dictates priority discharge summary, provides postdischarge telephone follow-up with patient)
- Rounds on LTAC patients
- Participates in the management of observation unit patients
- Provides patient education and management of specific disease states (e.g., diabetes)
- Shares patient care duties with clinical director (e.g., allowing administrative time for the director)

Assign a primary supervisor to the NPC, such as the hospitalist clinical director, but realize that there must be an immediate supervisor available whenever the NPC is working. Every hospitalized patient must be under the care of (and seen by) a physician per federal law. Regarding billing for NPC services, most practices bill according to Medicare's shared-visit rule, where joint NPC–physician visits are billed under the physician's billing number at 100% of the allowable rate [16]. Under this rule, the hospitalist must provide "face-to-face time" with the patient in addition to supervising the NPC.

A list of pros and cons may be created regarding utilization of NPCs in many of these activities. We will explore a few of these activities to illustrate this point.

- For example, NPCs are often positioned in the emergency department (as the hospitalist admission screener) to expedite the patient's admission into the hospital. This may hasten the patient's stabilization as well as avoiding bottlenecks in the emergency department. This placement also improves the efficiency of hospitalist physicians, allowing them to focus on established patients in the hospital.

- Conversely, most physicians prefer to admit their own patients, so they can become familiar with the clinical and psychosocial history contributing to an appropriate treatment plan. If the initial history and physical examination is performed by the NPC screener in the emergency department, it is probable that the patient will have another exam (by the attending hospitalist physician) during the first visit. This can become unsettling if the patient came into the hospital via the emergency department. In this scenario the emergency department provider would perform an examination prior to involving the admission screener. Therefore, the patient would have three examinations in short order! This inconvenience would be compounded further if the patient was transferred to the emergency department from the PCP's office and/or if residents were involved (yet an additional one or two examinations).

- NPCs may also be deployed as the discharging hospitalist. If they serve in this role for all hospitalist patients, this can free up the physicians to care for critically ill patients and/or see more patients. This will increase physician availability and productivity, allowing the program to expand its census. Having someone dedicated to this process may also improve discharge planning efficiency.

- On the other hand, if a provider other than the attending physician plans and coordinates the discharge, it may create a breakdown in continuity of care at one of the most crucial periods in the hospitalization. The discharging provider may not be aware of all aspects of the case and could neglect something significant. This may result in medication errors, failure to schedule follow-up studies or appointments, failure to transmit essential clinical information to the PCP, and/or failure to coordinate community/home services, to name a few problems.

11.3   PROGRAM POLICIES AND PROCEDURES

Development of a comprehensive practice management plan will provide your hospitalist program with both the necessary tools and structure to operate both efficiently and effectively. A comprehensive plan has several components that address the organizational, operational, financial, and clinical aspects of the program. Those components that the candidate may wish to discuss include (but are not limited to) the policy and procedure manual, staffing and scheduling protocol, billing protocol, performance scorecard, marketing plan, and the operational chain of command. Many programs have a short- and long-term strategic plan which may be discussed briefly with the candidate as well (see Section 11.5). Having these elements in place will support your physicians, allowing them to provide high-quality cost-effective medical care while accomplishing the program's objectives. A thriving program imparts practice stability and ultimately, job security for its physicians.

Share your practice management plan with potential hires. The plan will describe your organizational philosophy and practice culture. It also serves as an excellent recruitment tool, illustrating that the program is well managed and efficient. A well-run and fully functional program should allow the physician to thrive both clinically and financially. The goal is for the candidate to appreciate this fact and commit to your program. Next, we examine topics worthy of discussion during recruitment.

The Practice Manual

Outline the key operational principles of the practice that are found in the policy and procedure manual. The objective is to provide the candidate with an idea of your program's culture and modus operandi, not to review the manual in minute detail. Share the program's mission, vision, and objectives. Discuss the program's hours of service and rounding protocols (e.g., morning and afternoon rounds, evening check-out). Review the program's scheduling policies, including nighttime, weekend, and holiday coverage. Discuss briefly communication protocols, admission and discharge protocols, and physician coding and billing responsibilities.

11.4   PRACTICE SUPPORT

Candidates will be interested to learn about the systems that are in place to assist them in their job. Discuss the practice management tools that your program utilizes to support both physician and program success. These tools may include data-tracking systems, communication systems (e.g., Blackberries, PDAs, electronic medical records), concurrent coding and chart review, as well as educational sessions for the physicians. The educational sessions may address, for example, effective communication, conflict management and resolution, medico-legal risk, pay-for-performance measures, and customer service. These sessions may be complemented with other educational initiatives listed in Exhibit 11.5. Implementation of a sound practice management plan (e.g., one that supports physician performance and professional growth) will provide your program with a recruitment and retention advantage over competing programs.

Exhibit 11.5   Education Initiatives

There are many educational strategies (short of a Master's degree) that support hospitalist development as a leader of your program and/or as a leader within the sponsoring hospital. These strategies include:

- Leadership development conferences
- Administrative development conferences
- Business and accounting workshops
- Mentoring programs
- Development of a leadership tract within the hospital

11.5   STRATEGIC PLANNING

Short- and long-term strategic planning is crucial to the success of your hospitalist program. During the strategic process your program will analyze its strengths, weaknesses, opportunities, and threats. This process allows your practice to be proactive rather than reactive. For example, it may assist your program in developing a plan to address communication problems with PCPs: improving continuity of care, clinical outcomes, and PCP satisfaction. From the nonclinical perspective, it may contribute to identification of business partners and business opportunities.

Optimally, strategic planning should involve joint initiatives between the hospitalist practice and the sponsoring hospital. Joint initiatives can take many forms. In some instances, a weekend is dedicated to joint planning between the hospitalists and the hospital administration. This retreat may occur off hospital grounds so that all participants can be focused and engaged in the planning process. Strategic planning may also occur throughout the year via joint quarterly meetings between the hospitalist group and the hospital administrator overseeing the program. On a smaller level, monthly meetings may take place between the hospitalist clinical director and the hospital administrator. The take-home message is that collaboration between your program and the sponsoring hospital is essential to everyone's success.

Collaboration between the hospital and your hospitalist program should include the identification of common objectives and aligning incentives. Once the objectives are identified, a plan can be developed that allows all stakeholders to accomplish their goals. Hospital administration can support the process by promoting the hospitalist program both within the hospital and community as well as by providing the program with the tools necessary to succeed. Administration's support will empower the hospitalists as leaders within the institution and with the medical staff. Hospitalist providers may empower themselves within the institution by serving as a resource to the hospital staff (see Exhibit 11.6). The following examples illustrate the benefits of joint strategic planning.

- In 2009, hospital X (the sponsoring hospital for your hospitalist group) has listed as one of its goals a commitment to grow their orthopedic surgery program (with the long-term goal of establishing itself as an orthopedic center of excellence). One of your program's goals in 2009 is to increase market share within hospital X. During the strategic planning process, hospital X and your

Exhibit 11.6   Hospitalist Initiatives with the Hospital Staff

The hospitalist program can serve as a resource for the hospital staff in many ways. This will benefit both the hospital and hospitalist staff. In doing so, the physicians will improve the visibility of the hospitalist program and potentially their standing within the hospital hierarchy. The following is a short list of initiatives in which hospitalist providers can participate.

- Nursing educational sessions
- Participate on the utilization management committee
- ACLS training
- Code blue team training and participation
- Rapid-response team training and participation
- Teaching residents and students

hospitalist program decide to develop a preoperative clinic for those patients traveling to the hospital from outlying communities for orthopedic surgery. Your program guarantees preoperative clearance for all of these patients regardless of the time of day (e.g., 24/7 services). In return, hospital X agrees to subsidize your program an amount equivalent to one FTE, so that an additional hospitalist can be added to your practice. Thus, the planning process results in a win–win situation both for your program and for the hospital. Additional beneficiaries include the patients in outlying communities requiring orthopedic surgery and the ortho-pedic surgeons at hospital X.

- In many institutions, hospitalists are placed on key medical staff committees because of their breadth of knowledge. Some hospital-ists assume medical staff leadership positions based on their stature within the hospital (and among the medical staff). Placing hospi-talists in strategic positions will enable them to move both the program's and hospital's agendas in the desired direction. For example, if a hospitalist is on the performance improvement com-mittee, he or she may lobby for development of evidence-based clinical guidelines. This will allow care to be standardized within the hospital, which may result in both improving the quality of patient care and clinical outcomes. If the hospitalists are incentiv-ized based on clinical outcomes, they will benefit. The hospital will benefit if readmission rates are decreased (particularly for Medicare patients) and because the hospital may achieve its goals regarding both pay-for-performance and core measures.

- The hospitalist is typically one of the most knowledgeable physicians (if not the most knowledgeable) on the medical staff regarding the systems and inner workings of the hospital. Consequently, hospitalist administrators and medical staff leaders desire hospitalist involvement regarding medical staff business so they may draw on their experiences and expertise. Accordingly, the hospitalist clinical director may have a seat reserved on the medical executive committee. In some hospitals, the hospitalist clinical director has a seat reserved on the hospital board as well.
- Finally, your program may work closely with the hospital to develop care delivery systems that will support teamwork, job satisfaction (for hospitalist and hospital staff), and clinical excellence. These systems are discussed in detail in the next section. In order to develop these systems and accomplish the goals there must be cooperation from the hospital as well as from your program. Although the hospital will incur the costs for most of these programs, they will also be the beneficiaries of them. The costs may include hospital staff time, physical resources (e.g., dedicated hospitalist space, communication devices), and utilization of the hospital's information systems.

11.6   COLLABORATIVE SYSTEMS OF CARE

Many strategies and tools can be developed by both the hospital and your program to support the hospitalist objectives, clinical excellence, and professional fulfillment. The collaborative systems may include development of interdisciplinary rounds, a hospitalist case management program, a pharmacy consultation service, information technology programs, physician communication systems, and hospitalist recruitment and retention support. In this section we explore all of these strategies and tools.

Interdisciplinary Hospitalist Rounds

Development of interdisciplinary hospitalist rounds can be an effective tool to enhance communication among all health team members, supporting both hospitalist objectives and high-quality clinical outcomes. Interdisciplinary rounds may involve participation of the following professionals: hospitalist physicians, nursing staff, social workers, case managers, pharmacists, physical therapists, occupational therapists, and speech therapists. These rounds may be held daily or they may occur once or twice each week. Typically, time limits are imposed (e.g., 1 or 2 minutes per patient) to ensure efficiency. When rounds are run effectively, they enhance communication and teamwork among all health team members. This will focus all members on a similar clinical endpoint.

There are several goals of interdisciplinary rounds. Most important, interdisciplinary rounds aim to maximize clinical outcomes. In addition, they support delivery of cost-effective medical care by directing resource utilization and potentially decreasing length of stay. Discharge planning is also enhanced, which may decrease the readmission rate for some chronically ill (e.g., "frequent flyer") patients. If these goals are accomplished, patient and family satisfaction should be improved as well.

Case Management Program

Development of a hospitalist case management program will support appropriate discharge planning. Establishing a hospitalist discharge team is the first step in this development. The discharge team may consist of a dedicated case manager (for the hospitalist program), a social worker, a pharmacist, and a nurse. The team should be charged with appropriately evaluating and meeting the patient's needs at discharge. The team goal is to develop an outpatient management plan that will decrease the likelihood of readmissions.

Effective discharge planning is initiated at the time of admission and should consist of an evaluation of appropriate home and community resources for the patient. An evaluation of the patient's home resources consists of assessing both the support and availability of family and friends to aid the patient. In addition, it may require assessment of the physical layout of the home if the patient experiences problems with ambulation or eyesight. Discharge planning may also include coordination of appropriate community resources, such as home health services, physical/occupational therapy, hospice services, and adult patient daycare. It may entail evaluation of the patient's financial resources, insurance coverage, and formulary status as well.

Medication reconciliation is another essential aspect of the discharge process. The case managers can be empowered to coordinate this process. The managers must ensure that the process is completed prior to patient departure and that all parties involved (e.g., the patient, family, PCP, specialists) are aware of the discharge medications. In addition, the hospitalist must attest to the discharge medications and acknowledge that the patient was educated about the medications (e.g., reason for taking the medication, dosing schedule, side effects, changes in medications and/or dosing). A pharmacist may also be involved in this process (this is discussed in the next section). This function (in addition to medication reconciliation upon admission) is important for patient care and fulfills the Joint Commission regulations.

The case manager can also be charged with coordinating the follow-up outpatient PCP office visit and transmitting all relevant information to the PCP upon discharge. This includes the admission history and physical report, the discharge summary, and any important inpatient studies or reports. In some institutions, managers phone the PCP office notifying them of the discharge. In some instances that may also be responsible for calling the patient 24 to 48 hours after discharge to answer questions regarding the discharge plan (in many instances, this call is placed by either a hospitalist physician or an NPC).

Pharmacist Consultation Services

A registered pharmacist may also be called upon to provide a consultation prior to discharge. He or she may review the discharge medications (i.e., dose, timing, reason for medication, potential interactions, potential side effects, etc.) with the patient and/or family. Discussion may also occur regarding any change in medication from the patient's home medications. Some hospitals bill for this consultative service.

Information Technology Programs

Development of information technology programs (and systems) can support the hospitalist program (and hospital) by providing data and feedback on both clinical and financial performance. These data programs may translate to a hospitalist performance scorecard and an accompanying hospitalist performance committee (discussed below). In addition, information technology programs may allow concurrent performance review of the core measures of the Joint Commission and the Centers for Medicare and Medicaid Services (CMS). This information is critical, especially in the age of value-based purchasing. Value-based purchasing monetarily rewards providers and hospitals for delivering efficient, high-quality medical care to patients (e.g., pay for performance).

The following is a brief historical review to provide the reader with the background of the evolution of Medicare's value-based purchasing program. The Deficit Reduction Act of 2005 authorized CMS to develop a value-based purchasing program for Medicare hospital services beginning in 2009. Congress specified that the plan should address the collection, reporting, and validation of quality data, the structure of value-based payments, and the public disclosure of hospital performance. CMS defined the following goals for the Medicare hospital value-based purchasing program:

- Improve clinical quality
- Reduce adverse events and improve patient safety
- Encourage patient-centered care
- Avoid unnecessary medical costs
- Stimulate investments in systems (e.g., information technology) and care management tools and processes that are effective in improving quality and/or efficiency
- Make performance results transparent to consumers

As part of this initiative, CMS has collaborated with quality- and patient safety–focused organizations such as the Joint Commission, the National Quality Forum (NQF), and the Hospital Quality Alliance (HQA). The CMS value-based purchase performance measures apply to three performance domains: clinical quality, patient-centered care, and efficiency. The monetary incentives focus on quality measures' performance. Organizations that do not meet specified performance benchmarks will lose reimbursement. Thus, it is essential for the sponsoring hospital and hospitalist program to forge a partnership dedicated to delivering both high-quality patient care and successful clinical outcomes. Hospitals that develop information technology systems allowing for concurrent core measure performance review will support both the delivery of high-quality medical care and financial reward (for the institution and hospitalist program).

Development of a hospitalist performance scorecard or dashboard is an excellent tool to analyze core measure performance as well as other vital financial and clinical data (for the hospital and hospitalist program). The purpose of creating a scorecard is to improve the quality of patient care, the efficiency (and cost-effectiveness) of medical care, and the bottom line of both the hospitalist program and the hospital. To accomplish these goals the data must be timely, accessible, accurate, and reproducible (a challenge for most institutions). The sponsoring hospital's information technology team is typically responsible for developing systems and processes to collect the data required. As stated in Section 6.2, the common sources of data are the hospital's clinical and financial information systems and the hospitalist program's billing data.

Selection of scorecard metrics is a dynamic process and should be reevaluated annually. The core measure performance metrics discussed previously should be monitored for obvious reasons. There are a variety of other metrics worth consideration (see Exhibit 6.1). In general, metric selection will be guided by the hospitalist program's objectives as well as the latest national quality and patient safety initiatives (endorsed by regulatory agencies such as the Joint Commission and quality organizations such as IHI and Leapfrog). Some programs select metrics that measure return on investment for the sponsoring hospital. Others select those metrics that evaluate areas in need of improvement. Obtaining hospitalist input during the development of performance measures will be valuable. What physician knows the hospital (and hospitalist program) systems and processes more intimately than the physicians themselves? Hospitalist participation will also facilitate physician buy-in to the hospitalist performance program.

The performance scorecard should be formatted to allow for analysis of individual hospitalist, hospitalist practice, and hospital performance. The report can be customized, but data should be obtained and the information shared on a monthly (if possible), quarterly, and year-end basis. Comparison to previous year's data (e.g., five-year historical data if available) is also valuable. The scorecard can be presented in a monthly, quarterly, and year-to-date format. It is helpful to create a year-end report as well, with comparison to previous years.

As mentioned previously, the scorecard data should be gathered for individual hospitalist providers and the practice as a whole. The data are typically compared to local and national peer group data if this information is available (see Section 6.4). The scorecard data must be analyzed thoroughly, and trends must be tracked. Your program may decide to share this information with the hospitalists in a nonblinded manner, depending on the culture of the practice. Nonblinding the data may create healthy competition, which may drive performance and productivity in a positive manner. On the other hand, it can create tension between people and may ultimately be counterproductive if physicians refuse to assist one another.

Analysis of these data will provide information relating to the clinical and financial performance of both the hospitalist practice and sponsoring hospital. Creation of a hospitalist performance team and committee will provide a forum to monitor this performance. The committee can also provide root-cause analysis: identifying safety-based, production-based, process-based, failure-based, and systems-based failures. It can subsequently identify effective solutions that prevent recurrence.

The work of the performance committee should be a collaborative process between the sponsoring hospital and the hospitalist practice. The team should consist of key members from each entity. Participants may include a hospital administrator, the chief medical officer/vice president of medical affairs, and representatives from the nursing, case management/social service, quality assurance/performance improvement, information technology, emergency, and pharmacy departments. It should also include the hospitalist administrator, clinical director, and practice manager.

Depending on the choice of metrics, the hospitalist performance team may analyze information regarding morbidity and mortality rates, clinical outcomes, readmission rates, resource utilization, and physician productivity, coding, and chart documentation. It may also analyze various hospital departments and systems affecting the institution's (and hospitalist program's) clinical and financial performance. The data analysis may have far-reaching implications. For example, it may provide feedback and recommendations affecting:

- Hospital departmental staffing or procedural problems (e.g., contributing to patient safety issues, throughput difficulties, discharge delays)
- Information technology problems (e.g., collecting accurate, reproducible, and timely data)
- Communication problems [e.g., with the EMR, medical record or transcription department, with transitions of care (see below)]
- Hospitalist program staffing and/or practice model (e.g., problems with provider availability, provider burnout, continuity of care, inefficient care, high ALOS, patient throughput)
- Hospitalist policies and procedures (e.g., communication with key stakeholders, patient rounding, discharge planning, scope of deliverable services, hours of service).

Ultimately, successful hospitalist programs work collaboratively with the sponsoring hospital to critically evaluate the systems and processes affecting both patient care and financial performance. These programs are adept at applying the information obtained to create systems that support the delivery of high-quality patient care and successful clinical outcomes. Information may also be applied to bolster financial solvency (for the program and hospital) and stakeholder satisfaction (e.g., patient/family, hospital staff, PCP and specialist physician, hospitalist physician).

Provider Communication Systems

Effective communication between the hospitalist program and key stakeholders in the integrated healthcare delivery system is essential to the success of the program. Effective hospitalist communication supports continuity and coordination of care, patient safety, and successful clinical outcomes. It also supports cost-effective medical care (e.g., avoids duplication of services) and user satisfaction (e.g., patient, referring physician, specialist physician, hospital staff).

There are key communication interfaces, referred to as *transitions of care*, during a patient's hospitalization experience. These transitions begin before the patient is officially admitted into the hospital and conclude well beyond the physical discharge of the patient. These transitions include the hand-off from PCP to hospitalist upon transfer to the hospital. They may occur multiple times each day: for example, during morning checkout rounds (between the nighttime and daytime hospitalist), during nighttime checkout rounds (between the daytime and nighttime hospitalist), and with a change in the attending hospitalist physician. The discharge interface is another critical transition of care. Effective communication during the transitions of care is crucial to patient safety, the delivery of high-quality patient care, and successful clinical outcomes.

Processes and systems that support communication during the transitions of care are crucial. These may involve development of communication protocols and utilization of communication systems. Effective communication is dependent on collaboration between the hospitalist program and the hospital. For example, the hospital must ensure that the history and physical and discharge summary are transcribed in a timely manner. The system must also identify the providers (e.g., PCPs, specialists, nursing home, home health agency) in need of this information and transmit the reports in a timely manner. Finally, outstanding studies and reports (at the time of discharge) must be transmitted to the appropriate physicians. If your sponsoring hospital utilizes an EMR, many of these concerns are obviated (to those physicians having access). In other instances your hospitalist program should work with the sponsoring hospital to develop systems of communication. For example, many hospitals utilize an automatic facsimile system to transmit reports.

Day-to-day communication can also be challenging for hospitalist programs. Some programs or their sponsoring hospitals provide communication devices such as PDAs, Blackberries, or cell phones to facilitate the process (e.g., between hospitalists, between hospitalist and other physicians, between hospitalist and nurses). Some programs utilize a voicemail system for communication with PCPs. In some instances, bedside telemedicine rounds are made by the hospitalist while the PCP watches from his or her office! In other instances, consultations with specialists are obtained via telemedicine (this technology is provided by the sponsoring hospital). Finally, some hospitals offer a secured Web site for physician access.

Hospital–hospitalist collaboration may also occur during other communication interfaces between the hospital staff and hospitalist patients. For example, if a hospitalist patient is admitted from the emergency department, the department staff can provide a hospitalist practice brochure to the patient and family. The nursing staff on the hospital wards can also provide the brochure if the patient was not admitted through the emergency department. In doing so, these departments are promoting your hospitalist program. Nursing staff, case managers, or unit secretaries can also transmit the hospitalist discharge sheet (if one exists) to the PCP at discharge.

Creation of a hospitalist practice users group is another tool that supports communication. The meeting is typically held in the hospital, and participants may include hospitalist physicians, PCP/referring physicians, specialists, and emergency department providers. In some instances a hospital administrator is present (particularly if there are problems with hospital systems, processes, or services) and in other situations, nursing personnel may attend. The users group serves as a forum to discuss clinical, administrative, operational, or communication concerns related to the program and/or hospital. It also provides an opportunity to present new policies or services offered within the hospitalist program. During this meeting, potential drawbacks may also be discussed and feedback solicited from key stakeholders. This forum may be viewed as a consensus-building tool.

In the end, effective strategic planning provides stability for your hospitalist program. The process may identify internal problems and/ or external threats. It may also identify opportunities for collaboration. When your program forges professional relationships with various stakeholders in your integrated healthcare network, hospitalist performance is supported. Ultimately, the goal of effective strategic planning is to provide access and efficient, high-quality medical care in a cost-effective manner, all while achieving high grades in customer (e.g., patient, referring provider) satisfaction.

Share your strategic planning process with the candidate. Discuss all of the professional partnerships that your program has forged with key stakeholders in the community. It will be an excellent way to illustrate the culture within your practice as well as the support that your program enjoys. Program stability (and the job security it imparts) will be at the top of most candidates' list in their search for the right hospitalist opportunity.

11.7   MARKETING THE PROGRAM

Development of a marketing plan will support growth of your program. Marketing can be accomplished in many ways. For example, creation of a Web site is a simple, yet effective means to market your program. The Web site, can include a link for patients to navigate and one for referring providers. When creating your Web site, state your program's philosophy, mission, vision, and objectives. List the hospitalist providers accompanied by a picture and brief biography (e.g., medical school, specialty, residency, board certification, clinical interests). This allows the reader to put a face with a name. In addition, consider posting both patient and referring provider satisfaction survey results. If your program (or a provider in your practice) has received an award or recognition, this should be posted as well. A recruitment link for potential hospitalist candidates would also be valuable and can include (along with the information listed above) program specifics, such as the schedule, practice model, and services offered.

Creation of a community outreach program is a simple, yet effective marketing tool. This includes development of marketing brochures with content similar to your Web site. In addition, plan an annual visit by the clinical director to each referring physician's office. During this visit the director can field questions, obtain feedback and suggestions, provide updates regarding new services and new providers, review transfer protocols (from the office into the hospital and from the hospital back into the community), and query the front office staff regarding obstacles to transfer a patient into the hospital. The visit also provides an opportunity to thank the referring physicians for their support. Marketing visits can also be made to offices in outlying communities to drum up new business. Finally, some hospitalist programs team with a hospital administrator and make joint marketing calls.

A hospitalist newsletter is another simple tool to market your program. It can be sent quarterly or semiannually to the medical staff, hospital departments, and referring providers in the community. It can provide information similar to the Web site but should also include updates from the previous newsletter. It is an excellent vehicle to introduce new policies as well as new providers. An annual hospitalist

166 PRACTICE MANAGEMENT STRATEGIES

program update with the hospitalist staff and with the medical staff will complement the newsletter.

Finally, a recruitment video is another excellent tool to market your program. In this case the content should be geared toward candidates you would like to attract into your program. Feature sound bites from key stakeholders (e.g., the hospitalist administrator, hospitalist clinical director, hospital CEO, nursing director, patients, referring physicians, prominent people in the community). Provide information regarding the practice, hospital, medical staff, and community. Include relevant content with the candidate's spouse and family in mind.

Discuss your marketing plan with the candidate during the site visit. This can occur when you review the program's current referral base and future plans for growth. Although sharing information about the plan may appear to be extraneous, it will provide the candidate with an idea of the program's future direction. The candidate may also appreciate his or her participation in the future promotion of a successful hospitalist program. Additionally, the discussion will convey that your program is highly functional, well organized, and stable. Marketing plans serve to support continued program growth and ultimately job security.

12 Targeting Program Leadership

It has been mentioned throughout the book that the culture of your practice will play a significant role in attracting a candidate and/or retaining physicians for the long term. Many factors contribute to practice culture, and one of the most crucial is program leadership. Having an effective leader sets a positive tone for the program. Conversely, ineffective leadership can lead to a dysfunctional program, physician discord, and ultimately provider turnover.

In addition to practice culture, physician job satisfaction and the opportunity for professional development contribute to long-term physician retention. In 2006, SHM published a white paper titled "A Challenge on Hospitalist Career Satisfaction," which addressed the challenges that accompanied the growth and popularity of this specialty. This paper presented the framework for hospitalist career satisfaction, focusing on hospitalist program leadership and the "four pillars of career satisfaction." It also addresses individual hospitalist assessment relating to job fit, values, and goal alignment.

In this chapter we explore program leadership, practice culture, professional development, and career satisfaction. We discuss how these factors influence both program success and physician retention. Development of a leadership tract within your practice may allow you to identify and groom future leaders of your program. It will also support effective program leadership, physician retention, and career development. The creation of educational programs that allow physicians to pursue their professional interests supports both job satisfaction and career growth while decreasing the likelihood for burnout.

12.1 ATTRIBUTES OF EFFECTIVE PROGRAM LEADERSHIP

There are many reasons why hospitalists should take responsibility and assume a leadership position in healthcare. For instance, hospitalists

Hospitalist Recruitment and Retention: Building a Hospital Medicine Program,
By Kenneth G. Simone
Copyright © 2010 Wiley-Blackwell

serve in many roles in their sponsoring hospital (see Section 3.2). They serve as clinicians, educators, researchers, change agents, patient advocates, and as a resource for both medical and hospital staff. As such, they have much to contribute in the development and refinement of a diverse set of systems affecting the healthcare organization. These systems involve the day-to-day delivery of clinical care. In addition, these physicians affect the financial performance of both the hospital and the hospitalist program. The operational, clinical, and business systems address appropriate resource management, hospital and hospitalist program operations, hospital throughput, and information technology (e.g., EMRs). Optimal systems promote quality and patient safety, education, and continuity of care.

In many instances, hospitalists are called upon to lead their medical staff. They are asked to assist in medical staff recruitment and retention, and thus play a crucial role in medical staff stability (their very presence serves as a stabilizing force). Hospitalists are also asked to make a significant contribution within the sponsoring hospital by serving in leadership roles such as president of the medical staff, quality assurance director, and/or chief of the medicine, pediatric, or family medicine department. Their reach extends into the community, as these physicians serve the outpatient referral network. By improving the PCPs' quality of life and allowing these outpatient doctors to focus their efforts in one venue (e.g., increase practice efficiency) they make the community an attractive place to practice for many physicians. This will have a positive impact on PCP recruitment and retention.

Hospitalist programs should be cognizant of the many leadership roles that their doctors assume throughout the hospital and community. Recruiting hospitalists who have experience working with hospital administrators (e.g., the "c-suite") as well as an understanding of the organizational, operational, and business dynamics of institutional medicine will support the financial and operational success of both the hospitalist program and sponsoring hospital. Recruiting hospitalists capable of leading clinical initiatives (e.g., patient safety, quality, disease management, service line development), interdisciplinary teams, and a medical staff will enhance patient care outcomes and support program success. Identification of a candidate who possesses leadership potential but lacks experience may also be valuable if appropriate systems are in place to mentor the physician.

What makes an effective leader? The answer will vary depending on who you ask. That is because there are many different theories and styles of leadership. Furthermore, the definition of effective leadership may change depending on the context. The following are examples of various leadership theories.

- *Trait theory.* This theory describes personality tendencies and behaviors associated with effective leadership. Proponents of this theory list drive (including motivation, tenacity, initiative, and achievement), leadership motivation, honesty, integrity, self-confidence, cognitive ability, and knowledge of business as key leader traits.

- *Situational theory.* This theory postulates that different situations require different leadership characteristics and that no pure leadership profile exists.

- *Contingency theory.* The contingency theory defines leadership styles associated with specific situations. It integrates components of the trait and situational theories. This theory was refined further into four models: the Hersey–Blanchard situational theory (addresses four leadership styles and four levels of follower development), the Fiedler model (defines two leadership types: relationship- and task-oriented leaders), the path–goal theory (identifies four leader behaviors: achievement oriented, supportive, directive, and participative), and the Vroom–Yetton or situational contingency theory (proposes that the same leader could rely on different group decision-making methods, depending on the specific circumstances of each situation).

- *Transactional and transformational theories.* A *transactional leader* is empowered to lead the group in various tasks and to reward or punish the team's performance. The leader is also responsible to train, evaluate, and develop corrective action plans for suboptimal performance. A *transformational leader* serves as a team motivator to enhance both effective and efficient performance. The leader focuses on the big picture and utilizes a chain of command to accomplish the tasks. Transformational leaders are good communicators and are highly visible.

- *Functional theory.* This theory proposes that a leader's ultimate responsibility is to promote organizational effectiveness and cohesion. It is thought that the leader provides five functions to support performance: organizing subordinate activities, intervening in the group's work, teaching/coaching subordinates, motivating people, and monitoring the environment. Specific leader behaviors include role clarification, setting performance standards, holding people accountable, and expressing concern and/or support for subordinates.

- *Behavioral and style theories.*   These theories evaluate leadership styles and behaviors of successful leaders. It looks at various management styles, including (but not limited to):
  - *Laissez faire.* The leader is not involved in decisions and work, and rarely praises: may be effective with highly experienced employees who need little supervision.
  - *Authoritarian.* The leader makes decisions on his or her own, demands strict compliance to his or her orders, is detached from work activities, offers praise or criticism: appropriate for employees needing close supervision.
  - *Bureaucratic.* The leader is very structured, there is no exploration of new ways to problem solve, and the process is slow paced. A bureaucratic leader is appropriate for organizations looking to ensure quality, increase security, and decrease corruption, such as banks, universities, hospitals, and government.
  - *Democratic.* Collective processes and group perspectives are obtained. The leader provides technical advice, but members may decide the division of labor and provide objective feedback. This technique minimizes resistance and intolerance, which is a strength of this style, but the decision-making process is slow, which creates a problem when a plan of action is needed quickly.
  - *Charismatic.* The leader leads by infusing energy and enthusiasm into the team; he or she has magnetism. If team or project successes are attributed to the leader and not the team, these leaders may become a risk to move on to new, advanced opportunities.
  - *People oriented.* The leader supports, trains, and develops personnel to comply with effectiveness and efficiency; increases job satisfaction and interest in the job.
  - *Task oriented.* Focuses on the specific task of each employee to achieve goals. The method requires close supervision and control to achieve expected results; similar to the authoritarian style in that the leader is not involved in team needs.

A recent study by Christine Taylor and co-workers, "Exploring Leadership Competencies in Established and Aspiring Physician Leaders: An Interview-based Study," concluded that knowledge, people skills (also referred to as emotional intelligence), organizational altruism (e.g., understanding of and dedication to the institution), and vision were characteristics of effective leaders [17]. Integrity and the ability to engage, inspire, and empower others were other core leadership competencies that were mentioned. The authors raise the question of whether leadership is innate or can be learned.

If you explore the Internet in search of essential leadership qualities, traits, or characteristics, you will find additional definitions and varied descriptions. For example, one noted leader described five essential leadership traits as follows: A leader should have positive energy (to effect change); he or she should have edge (e.g., courage to make difficult decisions); a leader must execute (e.g., get the job done); he or she must have passion; and a leader must energize (e.g., inspire people). This notable leader was none other than Jack Welch, former chairman and CEO of General Electric Company. The following are insights (quotes) from other great leaders:

- "The task of the leader is to get his people from where they are to where they have not been." Henry Kissinger
- "Leadership is the art of getting people to do what you want them to do because they want to do it." Dwight Eisenhower
- "Obstacles are those frightful things you see when you take your eyes off your goal." Henry Ford
- "Outstanding leaders go out of their way to boost the self-esteem of their personnel. If people believe in themselves, it's amazing what they can accomplish." Sam Walton
- "There is no limit of what can be accomplished when no one cares who gets the credit." John Wooten
- "To solve big problems you have to be willing to do unpopular things." Lee Iacocca
- "Leadership and learning are indispensable to each other." John F. Kennedy

12.2 MENTORING POTENTIAL LEADERS

When your program identifies a potential leader among the ranks, it is both time and money well spent to groom this person. As mentioned in Section 2.9, hospitalist programs may experience considerable turnover. Thus, it is prudent to have "ready to lead" physicians available either to direct your program or to spearhead initiatives overseen by the hospitalist practice (e.g., serve as the director for quality assurance, the observation unit, the LTAC unit, the hospitalist residency tract or fellowship program) in the event of physician turnover. Development of a leadership mentor program should be based on the following fundamental tenets at a minimum:

- Identify aspiring leaders [e.g., these persons pursue professional and personal growth, see the big picture, are driven, exhibit excellent business sense, analyze and utilize data in the decision-making process, balance opposing forces (e.g., clinical versus business aspects of medicine, administrative versus provider agendas), search for new ideas, and have integrity].
- Identify established leaders (e.g., these people are competent, well respected, experienced, excellent teachers) in your community who are willing to mentor potential leaders.
- Pair the aspiring leader with compatible mentor(s).
- Develop a curriculum consisting of a didactic program (multidimensional and interactive) complemented by practical training. The program should cover core leadership competencies (established during creation of the mentor program and standardized for all aspiring leaders) by your mentor program leaders. Consider providing a C-I-A approach as part of the process [18]. *Concepts* can represent research-based principles and/or practical ideas that are applicable to the specific situation. *Illustration* refers to examples of what others have done and may include written case studies of successful or unsuccessful results, live case studies, role playing, web-2 applications, and so on. The participants learn by seeing how ideas were actually implemented (see below). *Application* reinforces concepts via personalization, as the aspiring leader adapts the lessons and illustrations to their situation.
- Provide CME funding for leadership courses (e.g., SHM Leadership Academy I and II) and hospitalist practice management courses.

Taylor et al. discuss curriculum design for programs desiring to enhance physician leadership skills [17]. They make the following observations and recommendations concerning curriculum considerations:

- Aspiring leaders' views differ somewhat from established leaders regarding the importance of organizational altruism and emotional intelligence. Therefore, it is important to share the traits that experienced leaders seek in evaluating a person for a leadership position.
- Train the aspiring leader in emotional intelligence, strategic planning, and organizational awareness.

- Utilize role playing, case studies, debate, and so on (e.g., participatory learning) to effect behavioral change among potential leaders. The literature supports interactive learning techniques to enhance learning and physician leadership development.
- Provide instruction regarding strategies for dealing with groups and mastery of specific bodies of knowledge (such as finance, regulatory issues, and legal issues). Provide training in networking skills, planning skills, and organizational planning. These various leadership characteristics were identified as "most teachable" (versus innate characteristics).

Aspiring leaders may ask: What are the keys to leadership success? The single most important key according to Ann Golden Eglè (a master certified coach who works with high-level executives, entertainers, and athletes) is the *presence* that a leader projects. According to Eglè presence consists of eight factors:

- Focus (e.g., commitment to long-term plan)
- Intellect (e.g., ability to analyze an issue from multiple perspectives)
- Charisma (e.g., ability to be intense, yet empathetic)
- Communication skills (e.g., communication style)
- Passion (e.g., enthusiastic)
- Culture fit (e.g., in tune with the organization's values and vision)
- Poise (e.g., maintains composure in all situations)
- Appearance (e.g., dresses the part)

Other keys to leadership success include leading by example, being a good listener, and being decisive.

12.3   LEADERSHIP VERSUS MANAGEMENT

Many people believe that leadership and management are synonymous, while others believe that management is a subset of leadership. The argument comes from the fact that leadership and management are similar. Depending on the definition you use, these terms may be considered the same or dissimilar. For the purposes of this book, management will be considered a subset of leadership. According to John Kotter, a professor at the Harvard Business School who many regard as an authority on leadership and change, leadership has been in existence for centuries whereas the concept of management has been advanced only in the last century. Development of the management concept is believed to have occurred in part as a result of the industrial revolution.

To clarify this point further, let us define leadership. According to BusinessDictionary.com, in its essence leadership in an organizational role involves (1) establishing a clear vision; (2) sharing (communicating) that vision with others so that they will follow willingly; (3) providing the information, knowledge, and methods to realize that vision; and (4) coordinating and balancing the conflicting interests of all members or stakeholders. What is the definition of management? According to BusineessDictionary.com, *management* is organization and coordination of the activities of an enterprise in accordance with certain policies and in achievement of clearly defined objectives. Management is often included as a factor of production along with machines, materials, and money. As a discipline, management comprises of the interlocking functions of formulating corporate policy and organizing, planning, controlling, and directing the firm's resources to achieve the policy's objectives.

Management and leadership activities commonly interface and allow for a reciprocal relationship. For example, when managers oversee employees so that the employees may meet their objectives, they are leading; thus, effective managers should possess leadership skills. When leaders are involved in planning or staffing, for example, they are actively managing; thus, effective leaders must display management capabilities. Although there is overlap, Warren Bennis delineated 12 distinctions between these two entities (see Exhibit 12.1). Comparing and contrasting these two groups will allow your program to choose an appropriate fit for a specific task it needs to accomplish. It will also provide insight concerning the type of candidate you wish to hire based on the needs and future direction of your program. For example, if your program is anticipating expansion through the creation of an observation unit for the sponsoring hospital (e.g., requiring additional physicians for the practice), hiring a physician with managerial skills would be an appropriate choice. On the other hand, if your program is expanding to another hospital (possibly in another state), recruitment of a physician with leadership skills would be an appropriate choice to build and direct the program.

In terms of day-to-day task comparisons between the manager and leader one may describe the manager as creating order, stability, and structure, while the leader elicits change, advancement, and growth.

Exhibit 12.1   Differences Between Managers and Leaders

Warren Bennis demonstrated the major differences between leadership and management in 1989 [19]. He made 12 distinctions concerning the functional roles of managers and leaders.

Managers	Leaders
Administer	Innovate
Imitate	Originate
Maintain	Develop
Focus on systems	Focus on people
Do things right	Do the right thing
Have short-term perspective	Have long-term perspective
Emulate the good soldier	Are their own person
Ask how and when	Ask what and why
Rely on control	Inspire trust
Eye the bottom line	Eye the horizon
Copy	Show originality
Accept the status quo	Challenge the status quo

Managers plan, budget, organize, and control for specific activities such as resource allocation, development of policies and procedures, recruitment, and performance improvement. These individuals set timetables, establish agendas, and develop incentives. Leaders, on the other hand, establish direction, motivate, and inspire others. They are excellent communicators and empower individuals to perform to their best abilities. Leaders create strategic plans (short and long-term), build consensus and coalitions, and create a common organizational vision.

Hospitalist leaders must possess both management and leadership skills. For example, they are responsible for running hospitalist practice meetings, developing and implementing program policies and procedures, creating physician work schedules (including staffing shortage management), and monitoring (and acting upon) provider performance. In addition, they must develop and implement strategic initiatives, build consensus among the staff, as well as inspire, motivate, and empower the physicians. Hospitalist leaders must also apply their skills with other key stakeholders such as hospital administrators (e.g., the "c-suite"), the medical staff, and the hospital staff.

12.4   IDENTIFYING AND RECRUITING AN EFFECTIVE LEADER

Identification and recruitment of an effective physician leader for your program will be quite challenging. To succeed you must create the necessary tools and structure before embarking on the recruitment process. This entails creation of a clinical director job description (see Exhibit 12.2) and defining specific candidate selection criteria. In addition, it requires implementation of an effective candidate search and interview process, and perhaps most important, identification of the appropriate leadership style that fits the practice, medical staff, and hospital staff culture, and complements the administrative team (of the practice and sponsoring hospital). Choice of leadership style will also be influenced by the specific requirements of your program, taking into consideration both current and future needs.

Exhibit 12.2   Clinical Director Job Description

Development of a hospitalist clinical director job description is critical to this person's success. This document will provide the leader with your program's vision of his or her role and performance expectations. The director's job description should be based on the specific leadership needs of your program. It should define the specific job responsibilities and expectations (clinical, supervisory, and administrative). It should clearly delineate the organizational chain of command; addressing the director's accountability and scope of authority. The job description should be structured in a fashion similar to that of the other hospitalists. This includes specification about academic training, board certification, field of specialization, required knowledge, skills, and abilities, and previous employment experience.

The following example provides a multitude of concepts you should consider when creating the clinical director's job description:

- *Position summary*. Provide a brief description of the job responsibilities. For example, the summary should delineate the director's clinical, supervisory, leadership, and administrative responsibilities. It should clearly state that the director will support and promote the mission, values, and objectives of the hospitalist program (and hospital if employed by the hospital). It should also state that the physician is responsible for adherence to the program's policies, procedures, and strategic plan. Furthermore, the summary may indicate that the director is expected to formulate strategic plans and ensure attainment of the program's operating goals.

- *Essential job functions*
  - ○ Leadership responsibilities
    - ▪ Provide organizational leadership
    - ▪ Coordinate provider schedules, time-off requests, appropriate day-to-day staffing of program, etc.
    - ▪ Participate in leadership committees within the hospital (e.g., medical executive, peer review, utilization management, quality and patient safety, finance)
    - ▪ Participate actively in hospitalist recruitment (and long-term recruitment planning)
    - ▪ Provide oversight of the hospitalist orientation and mentoring program
    - ▪ Chair the hospitalist performance committee
    - ▪ Chair the hospital quality assurance committee (e.g., quality, patient safety, outcome initiatives)
    - ▪ Develop, participate in, and provide oversight of quality initiatives and the hospitalist incentive plan
    - ▪ Conduct monthly chart reviews when necessary
    - ▪ Represent the program with key stakeholders (e.g., hospital administration, medical staff, hospital staff, patients, families), including mediation when necessary
    - ▪ Participate actively in program marketing
    - ▪ Participate in development of the program's short- and long-term strategic plan
    - ▪ Identify program opportunities and assist in development of new practice service lines
    - ▪ Provide operational leadership: oversee hospitalist practice operations (nonclinical and clinical)
    - ▪ Provide leadership and act as an educator for the providers (e.g., customer service, time management, productivity strategies, resource management, cost-effectiveness)
    - ▪ Monitor referral network
    - ▪ Provide managed care leadership: contracting, development of pay-for-performance initiatives (including monitoring, managing, and reporting)

- ○ Clinical responsibilities: same as for other hospitalist physicians
- ○ Administrative responsibilities: same as for other hospitalists. In addition, provide reports and evaluations relating to the various roles and responsibilities of the clinical director.
- *Supervisory responsibilities.* The clinical director is responsible for supervising all clinical staff, residents, interns, and medical students, if applicable. The director must also provide oversight of the nonclinical staff and practice operations.
- *Reporting structure.* State clearly the organizational chain of command: for example, who reports to the clinical director and to whom the clinical director reports.
- *Job requirements and expectations.* Define clearly hospitalist requirements and expectations. For example, he or she must:
  - ○ Have an unrestricted medical license to practice medicine in the state or states where your program is located.
  - ○ Be credentialed and privileged to practice medicine at the sponsoring hospital.
  - ○ Work whatever the number of specified hours per week your program requires and the number of call hours per week (if your program has call responsibilities).
  - ○ Provide necessary administrative time each week to complete medical records (as consistent with medical staff bylaw requirements) and all paperwork in a timely manner.
  - ○ Complete the specified number of CME hours (annually or biennially) as required by the medical staff bylaws and state licensure board.
- *Knowledge, skills, and abilities required.* Address the core competencies that a hospitalist clinical director must possess for your program. This should include:
  - ○ Provide program leadership in all areas that serve to improve patient outcomes, position the practice as the premier care giver within the hospital and medical community, and advance the field of hospital medicine.
  - ○ Possess the ability to consensus build, motivate, train, and work with staff
  - ○ Possess the ability to establish and maintain strong line of communication with key stakeholders (e.g., patients/families, hospitalist providers, referring PCPs, specialists, nurses, hospital administration).

- ○ Possess the ability to develop treatment plans, manage patients, and develop discharge plans for each patient.
- ○ Possess in-depth coding and chart documentation knowledge.
- ○ Possess knowledge of both the hospitalist and integrated healthcare delivery network system.
- ○ Possess the ability to develop and implement new systems, policies, and procedures.
- ○ Possess the ability to demonstrate strong analytical skills and develop improvement plans concerning the hospitalist's utilization of resources, productivity, clinical performance, and financial performance.
- ○ Possess the ability to affect patient outcomes, core measure performance, and pay-for-performance outcomes through a systems approach.
- ○ Possess the ability to participate in development of evidence-based clinical protocols.
- ○ Possess managed care knowledge regarding risk contracts (e.g., quality and safety initiatives, resource utilization).
- ○ Possess skill in establishing and maintaining effective and collaborative working relationships with the medical staff, referring providers, hospital staff, and the community.
- ○ Possess the ability to supervise and manage the hospitalist physicians and clerical personnel in a professional and constructive manner.
- ○ Possess skills to coordinate provider scheduling.
- ○ Possess the ability to supervise NPCs, residents, interns, and medical students (if applicable).
- *Typical working conditions.* Describe the typical work environment (both office and hospital) and discuss potential exposures (e.g., communicable diseases, toxic substances, medicinal preparations, needles, body fluids). Delineate travel requirements.
- *Typical physical demands.* Describe the typical physical activities and skills required (e.g., sitting, standing, reaching, lifting patients with assistance, normal range of hearing and eyesight, hand–eye coordination, manual dexterity to operate computer keyboard and telephone)
- *Education and work experience required.* Address the following:
  - ○ Work experience required (e.g., three to five years as a practicing hospitalist or in private practice)

- Leadership experience required, which may be defined in several ways, for example:
  - Previous experience as a hospitalist clinical director highly preferred
  - Three to five years of experience in a leadership position (or specifically as a hospitalist clinical director)
  - M.B.A., M.H.A., or M.P.H. recommended (or required)
- Educational experience required (e.g., must be a graduate of an accredited allopathic/osteopathic medical school)
- Training experience required [e.g., must complete an internal medicine, family practice, or medicine–pediatrics residency (if an adult program) or a pediatric residency (if a pediatric program)]
- Areas of expertise required may address the following:
  - Must have experience leading pay-for-performance, quality, and patient safety initiatives
  - Must have experience working in a complex integrated health-care delivery system
  - Must have experience negotiating managed care contracts
  - Must have experience creating a program budget, proforma, business plan, and so on.
  - Must have experience with clinical protocol and guideline development, care management program development, and outcome measurement assessment development
  - Must have a solid knowledge base of current practices, methods, and procedures in hospitalist medicine
  - Must have excellent communication skills with peers, hospital personnel and patients; and knowledge of, and willingness to work within, a managed care environment
- Board certification requirements [e.g., must be board certified (as opposed to the other hospitalists, who may be board eligible)]
- Reference requirements (e.g., must have acceptable references from the director of the residency training program, physicians, hospital personnel, previous employers, and persons chosen by your program; references are difficult to assess for a number of reasons, and it may be beneficial in some instances to choose the reference)

Proceed with caution during the recruitment process, as there are many potential pitfalls (see Section 8.1). For example, the candidate's agenda may not be aligned with yours. Some candidates view a leadership position as an excellent opportunity to wind down a career (as counterintuitive as that may seem). Other candidates may be burned out from work on the "front line" and may be seeking solace in this role. Some applicants are attracted to the position because of their desire for power. Creating a process to sort this out vigorously is crucial for your program. Solicit effective and trusted leaders within the community to participate in the process. These people will be adept at screening candidates. Provide a checklist of selection criteria (with an accompanying scorecard) for all participants' utilization. This will guide an objective screening process (see Exhibit 12.3).

Exhibit 12.3   *The Clinical Director Selection Criteria Checklist*

The following is an example of selection criteria that your recruitment team can utilize to screen potential clinical director candidates. The checklist establishes an objective process allowing you to compare various candidates. This process, in essence, defines the necessary skills, knowledge, and professional experience that the clinical director must possess. The checklist addresses the specific attributes desired in a clinical director. In addition to using this checklist as a screening tool, it can be developed into an interview scorecard. The scorecard should also include all of the criteria that are utilized for nondirector candidates, such as appearance, interpersonal skills, practice compatibility, work ethic, long-term goals and dependability, clinical acumen, and previous experience (see Exhibit 9.5).

- *Leadership experience*
  - Medical practices
  - Medical staff
  - Hospital staff
  - Local community
  - Nationally
- *Leadership skills*
  - Ability to communicate effectively with subordinates and other stakeholders
  - Ability to represent and advocate positively for the practice with all stakeholders

- ○ Ability to motivate the staff and other stakeholders
- ○ Adept at change management
- ○ Ability to build consensus
- ○ Ability to teach and train
- ○ Ability to develop new and effective systems and process
- ○ Ability to manage the team's time
- ○ Ability to manage quality and regulatory initiatives
- ○ Ability to build customer base and build new services associated with the program
- *Leadership style*
  - ○ Your team must decide on appropriate and acceptable leadership characteristics and styles that complement both the practice and the hospital culture
- *Administrative experience*
  - ○ Effective program management
  - ○ Organizational leadership
  - ○ Executive leadership
  - ○ Collaborative processes with hospital administration
- *Business experience*
  - ○ Operational
    - Practice systems
    - Collaborative systems with other institutions
    - Ability to affect physician productivity and practice expenses positively
  - ○ Service line development
  - ○ Budgetary
  - ○ Fiscal responsibility
  - ○ Managed care
    - Pay-for-performance initiatives
    - Contracting
  - ○ Marketing
- *Ability to motivate and inspire*
- *Self-confidence*
- *Ability to evoke confidence*
- *Practice fit*
- *Commitment to the program for the long term*

Evaluate your program's leadership chain of command critically prior to initiation of your search. Ensure that the current structure is appropriate and make changes where needed. Evaluation of leadership infrastructure begs the following questions: Would a seasoned leader want to assume a central role in your organization? Do the clinical director's job description and your organizational structure allow the physician autonomy? Does the organization provide the required support for the operational, leadership, and administrative functions expected of the director? Does the candidate have an opportunity for professional growth and development? The answers to these questions will guide your recruitment process. For example, if the clinical director is accountable to multiple parties (e.g., hospitalist practice administration, practice shareholders or board members, hospital administration), he or she must be capable of balancing a variety of agendas. This structure may drive away an experienced candidate who may feel micromanaged under such conditions. On the other hand, it may provide the needed guidance and support for an inexperienced but promising leader. If your program's administrative and organizational support is limited (due to staffing or budgetary reasons, for example), selection of a seasoned leader who is self-directed and self-motivated would be a logical choice.

The recruitment team should also determine what leadership style(s) would be appropriate for the program. This decision involves consideration of many factors. The following is a sampling of the factors your program may consider:

- Current practice culture (e.g., Are the current physicians self-motivated? Productive? Team players? Are there disruptive physicians within the practice? Do the hospitalists support the program's mission and goals? Do they follow the program's policies and procedures? Are they integrated within the medical staff? How are the hospitalists perceived in the hospital and community?)

If there are problems within the program, strong consideration should be given to the selection of an experienced leader. The appropriate candidate for dysfunctional practices may be the transactional leader, the authoritarian, or one whose leadership style is similar to the leader described in the functional theory (see Section 12.1). When buy-in is problematic among the hospitalists, the people-oriented leadership style may improve job satisfaction and the hospitalist's compliance with the program's policies, procedures, and objectives.

- Current practice performance (e.g., Do the physicians practice evidence-based medicine? Are the morbidity, mortality, and readmission rates appropriate? What about clinical outcomes? Do the physicians practice efficient and cost-effective medicine? Are they focused on the business aspects of medicine (coding, chart documentation, billing, etc.)? How are patient, referring physician/ medical staff, nursing, and emergency department satisfaction with the program?

If your program has problems with clinical performance, consider recruiting a systems- and processes-oriented director, an academic leader, or one who has extensive experience overseeing quality initiatives. If your program falls short on the business and financial side, a leader who possesses extensive business experience may be the proper fit. A transformational or charismatic leader may an appropriate choice if there are customer service issues.

- Desired practice culture and performance (based on the short- and long-term strategic plan of the program, for example; the desire to assume greater responsibility in the hospital, develop additional services or contract them, start a teaching program, forge a collaborative relationships with outlying hospitals, etc.)

If your program is expanding its service line, a democratic-style leader may be an excellent choice. These leaders build consensus and support, which will minimize pushback from the hospitalists. A task-oriented, innovative, or entrepreneurial leader would also be an ideal choice, as would a person adept at marketing.

- Administrative culture (e.g., hospitalist administration, hospital administration)
- Hospital culture (e.g., medical staff, nursing staff, key departmental leaders)

The answers to these and other questions will help focus your recruitment team and their recruitment efforts concerning the leadership type desired. As demonstrated above, there is no right or wrong leadership style (for the most part). Some situations warrant selection of decisive, action-oriented leaders, whereas others may necessitate more passive or process-driven leaders. During the recruitment process it will be valuable to query people who have worked for or with the candidate as a means of learning about his or her leadership style. It will also be beneficial to ask the candidate situational or behavioral descriptive questions to focus on performance in past circumstances. This line of questioning will provide information about the physician's ability to analyze a problem and create an optimal solution.

Your search for the appropriate leader will also be influenced by both the type of hospitalist program and the services offered. For example, academic hospitalist programs require a leader who is experienced (or knowledgeable) with the organizational structure, operation, and administration of a residency program. Experience in teaching, training, and research will be beneficial.

Finally, develop strategies that will support the effective performance and retention of your hospitalist clinical director. For example, your hospitalist practice must ensure that appropriate systems and programs are in place that allow the director to accomplish his or her day-to-day responsibilities. Development of a leadership mentor program for your clinical director will support success and be an excellent retention tool as well. In addition, aligning your program's goals with the directors will be beneficial. This will necessitate discussion about the short- and long-term vision and objectives of the practice while soliciting feedback and input from the director. Your program should also clearly define the program expectations, the director's accountabilities, and should share with the director the anticipated time commitment for administrative and leadership responsibilities. Keep in mind that unmet expectations and poor cultural fit within the practice may result in turnover.

Finally, your hospitalist practice must ensure that systems and programs are in place to position the new clinical director for success and support retention. Development of a leadership mentoring program for your clinical director will support success and be an excellent retention tool as well. In addition, clearly define both program expectations and the director's accountabilities. Share with the director the anticipated time commitment for administrative and leadership responsibilities. Provide the short- and long-term vision and objectives of the practice. Elicit feedback and input from the director and align your program's goals with the directors. Keep in mind that unmet expectations and poor cultural fit within the practice may result in turnover.

Programs that support professional autonomy and provide directors with authority are more likely to attract and retain exceptional leaders for the long term. The same can be said for organizations that value diversity and allow active participation by the director in the program's operations (e.g., budget process, service line development, program marketing). In many instances, clinical directors have left their program because they were never empowered to lead or direct.

12.5   PRACTICE CULTURE AND CAREER SATISFACTION

As noted earlier, in 2006, SHM published a white paper entitled "A Challenge on Hospitalist Career Satisfaction" that serves as an excellent resource concerning hospitalist career satisfaction. The paper provides tools and strategies to support job satisfaction and avoid physician burnout. It presents strategies that leaders can use to influence four areas (or pillars) that affect job satisfaction: reward recognition, workload schedule, autonomy/control, and community/environment. It also addresses the individual hospitalist's role in career satisfaction, which includes finding the right job. The paper lists four areas of job control that contribute to career satisfaction: task control, decision/organizational control, physical environment control, and resource control. The following sections are based on this white paper, with suggested applications that will support recruitment and retention of high-quality hospitalist physicians.

Pillar 1: Reward and Recognition

Employees in any occupation desire recognition and reward for their work and performance. In your practice there are ample opportunities to accomplish this. Systems must be in place to evaluate the physicians and practice as a whole objectively before you can recognize and reward performance appropriately. For example, physicians can be evaluated based on their clinical performance (e.g., quality initiatives and outcomes), productivity (RVUs), and financial performance (e.g., appropriate resource utilization, appropriate coding, timely and accurate bill submission). In addition, they can be rewarded based on citizenship (e.g., willingness to help others and/or go above and beyond expected duties, take time to teach and instruct hospital staff), participation in non-clinical activities (e.g., committee work, serve in leadership roles such as department chief or medical staff president, assist in creation of clinical pathways), and teamwork (e.g., assist fellow hospitalists when the need arises, such as taking an extra admission, taking extra call during times of unexpected illness or if the practice is understaffed). Performance-specific indicators may change annually based on your program's specific needs, goals, and previous accomplishments (individual and practice). Hospitalist performance can be evaluated quarterly, through implementation of an incentive plan, and/or annually. It may also occur through the use of satisfaction surveys. These topics are covered elsewhere in the book.

Hospitalists may be recognized and rewarded both on an individual basis and as a group. Individual rewards are typically financial in nature (e.g., reflected in salary, bonus, additional paid time off). This topic was discussed in detail in Chapter 6. Rewards may also be what the white paper terms *social* (e.g., expression of appreciation by fellow hospitalists, colleagues, hospital staff, hospital administration, patients), and/or *intrinsic* (e.g., satisfaction from personal work performance, helping others, growing professionally). When the medical staff, outpatient referring providers, and/or (sponsoring) hospital administration acknowledge the work performed by the hospitalists (and the value it provides to the medical community), it supports hospitalist job satisfaction. It accomplishes this by making the hospitalist team and individual physicians feel appreciated and respected for the job they perform. Respect and recognition by the stakeholders will contribute to a gratifying work environment for the hospitalists.

The hospitalists may also be recognized and rewarded as a practice. When the hospitalists are rewarded as a group, the sponsoring hospital, for example, may provide the practice with additional administrative support, physical space, subsidy, and/or equipment. Other forms of rewards may include appointment of a hospitalist to an open leadership position or key committee (e.g., executive, finance), which will enhance the program's stature and influence within the hospital. Acknowledgment of program accomplishments may also come in the form of recognition within the hospital (or hospitalist) newsletter. The take-home message is one in which the hospitalists must feel valued by the stakeholders (e.g., referring physicians, hospital administration, the nursing staff, the emergency department).

Pillar 2: Workload/Schedule

Hospitalist workload can be measured in several ways. This includes work volume and work intensity (e.g., ADC, number of admissions, number of discharges, number of consultations, acuity of patients), and type of work (e.g., patient care, teaching, administrative work, research), which are easy to measure. It also includes categories that are more difficult to measure, which SHM's white paper terms *time pressure* (e.g., the need to get work done in a specified timeframe), *interruptions* (e.g., unexpected beeper or telephone calls, unexpected emergencies), and *work variability* (regarding volume, intensity, and pressure). It is important to assess workload so that your program can provide appropriate staffing and support.

Because of its unpredictable nature management of physician workload is one of the most difficult challenges that confront every hospitalist program. Your program can develop several strategies to address this challenge and avoid burnout and job dissatisfaction. For example, implementation of a schedule and practice model that is tailored to your program's needs is very important (see Chapter 5). This involves both assessment and definition of the program's clinical and nonclinical physician responsibilities (e.g., program scope of services), work volume and intensity, physician productivity, and operational needs (e.g., clinical and nonclinical staffing). Your program may modify its schedule based on the findings. For example, you may change the length of each shift, the number of consecutive days worked, the number of consecutive days off (e.g., recovery time), and the night call schedule. The program may also decide to implement a physician patient cap (but not a practice cap) protecting individual physicians (and their patients) should their census approach an unworkable volume.

Implementation of an appropriate schedule and practice model also requires evaluation of both practice and institutional (e.g., hospital) systems that are currently in place to support the hospitalist program and physician performance. If the hospitalists believe that their ability to perform effectively is hindered by these systems, your program can develop systems that support physician efficiency and promote productivity. This may involve, for example, implementation of preprinted evidence-based clinical order sets, and utilization of NPCs within the practice to assist the hospitalist physicians. It may also involve a collaborative approach with the sponsoring hospital, such as the implementation of interdisciplinary patient rounds, development of a hospitalist case management program, and/or creation of a hospitalist discharge team.

Your practice can also develop programs to support physician wellbeing. For example, development of an employee assistance program can be valuable for the providers. This program can provide both an assessment of the physician's problems and assistance to deal with them. Assistance can be provided for a diverse range of problems, such as anger management, work relationship issues, emotional distress, depression and anxiety, substance abuse, family/personal relationship issues (e.g., marital difficulties), grief and bereavement, and financial or legal concerns. The program can also provide assistance regarding time management, stress management, communication skills, and job performance. Finally, some programs offer proactive prevention as well as health and wellness activities for their physicians.

Pillar 3: Autonomy/Control

Physician autonomy and sense of workplace control are important factors affecting both job satisfaction and burnout. The operative word is *sense*, because control is very subjective and relies on a person's perception. For example, when a physician feels that there are workplace obstacles affecting the execution of job responsibilities, stress and frustration typically result. The same is true if a physician believes that he or she is unable to modify various factors within the practice that affect work performance. Development of strategies to support an autonomous workplace and to empower the physicians will help prevent burnout and job dissatisfaction longitudinally.

Your program should be proactive concerning physician perceptions of workplace autonomy and job control. For example, mismatched expectations between the physician and hospitalist practice may occur if the job expectations were not communicated clearly during the recruitment and orientation process (and if the job description is vague). This can lead to physician alienation and control misperceptions which may ultimately result in job dissatisfaction and physician turnover. Create an orientation program (and follow-up periodically) to address workplace conditions, autonomy, and job control (see Chapters 8 and 9). In addition, make sure that the hospitalist job description clearly defines the job requirements, job expectations, clinical responsibilities, and administrative responsibilities.

In addition to these strategies, the hospitalist clinical director can be instrumental in empowering the physicians and ensuring an autonomous workplace. The director's leadership style will influence this. For example, if he or she leads in an authoritarian or bureaucratic manner, the other hospitalists may feel like they have no control or autonomy. If the director leads in a democratic manner or is people oriented (rather than task oriented), this will empower the physicians and foster both autonomy and a sense of job control. Additional strategies to support these goals include the implementation of a mentor program in the first year of employment as well as three-, six-, and 12-month meetings between the clinical director and the new physician to both obtain feedback and offer support and advice. This will allow the new physician to make suggestions on the work and practice environment. Finally, holding regular provider meetings between the clinical director and hospitalist physicians will be beneficial to obtain input and empower the physicians.

Evaluation of the hospital's role in autonomy and job control is important. For example, if the physicians do not have ready access to workstations, patient charts, or computer terminals, efficiency and performance may be affected (dedicated hospitalist office space and equipment is also necessary). In addition, the physicians should have access to nursing personnel, case managers, and social workers (hospitalist support staff is also necessary). Accessibility of clinical services and patient resources such as subspecialists, home health and hospice services, and LTAC units will also influence a physician's perceptions regarding control. When these systems and services are not in place, the clinical director must address this with the appropriate stakeholders. A proactive approach to avoid further problems involves placement of hospitalist physicians on key medical staff committees (e.g., executive, performance improvement, quality assurance, utilization management) and hospital committees (e.g., hospital board, capital expenditure–finance).

Pillar 4: Community/Environment

The fourth pillar refers to professional and interpersonal relationships within the "community." The white paper defines four communities: hospital, hospitalist, patient, and home. The *hospital community* refers to hospital administration, hospital staff, the emergency department, referring and nonreferring physicians, house staff, and medical students. The *hospitalist community* includes all members of the hospitalist practice, as well as relationships with other hospitalist practices and physicians. The *patient community* consists of patients, patient families, and the community served by the hospitalists and hospital. The *home community* refers to the "external" environment, including family and friends. All of these communities will have a significant bearing on physician well-being and job satisfaction.

Your program must analyze the expectations of all stakeholders (e.g., communities) interacting with the practice in order to assess the hospitalist work environment. The practice can assess whether inequalities exist regarding gender, race, sexual orientation, and so on. In addition, evaluation of both the hospital and hospitalist office environment regarding interpersonal and professional interactions will be extremely helpful. It is also important to assess communication and technological support within the workplace (and office).

If there are mismatched expectations with any stakeholders, strategies can be implemented to address this. For example, creation or improved distribution of a practice brochure and/or creation of a hospitalist Web site may be beneficial to educate the community (e.g., patients, families, hospital staff, medical staff, outpatient physicians). The brochure and Web site can provide information about the hospital-ist providers (e.g., training, degree, board certification, areas of inter-est), the hospitalist program (e.g., mission, vision, objectives, scope of service, access information), and practice protocols (e.g., admission, communication, rounding). Development of a marketing plan may serve to align everyone's expectations (e.g., the hospital, hospitalist, and patient communities). Creation of a users' group may be an excel-lent tool to improve relationships between key stakeholders within the hospital community.

Development of support technology to enhance communication across all communities will be helpful. Technological support may include utilization of computers, phone systems, voice mail, fax, and so on. Development of communication protocols may also be valuable. These protocols may address various communication problem points, such as the admission interface, when a patient is being transferred from one physician to another and at the time of patient discharge from the hospital. These protocols may also involve postdischarge telephone follow-up with the patient and/or family member. Finally, utilization of satisfaction surveys to query various stakeholders can be an excel-lent tool to ensure that expectations are aligned.

If dysfunction exists within the workplace, if there are problems with team chemistry, or if there's conflict among any community or group of persons, there must be appropriate intervention to resolve the situ-ation. If this doesn't occur, the consequences can be dire for workplace satisfaction for all stakeholders. A toxic work environment can lead to physician turnover, hospital staff turnover, a lapse in communication (among all stakeholders), poor clinical outcomes, and patient safety concerns. The intervention may require the involvement of human resource staff. This may necessitate the involvement of both the hos-pital and hospitalist administration, and/or require the utilization of consultants. It may also involve work on team building and group development.

Many organizations undertake team building (or organizational development) exercises to assist stakeholders in identifying and focus-ing on the common goals of the group and to instill "ownership" among all persons. Typically, the team undergoes a self-assessment process to assess its effectiveness, identifying both strengths and weaknesses. The team then develops strategies to improve performance and enhance teamwork. The process also involves recognizing obstacles that may confront the group and developing strategies and systems to overcome them. In the event no clear solution exists, which is a very realistic possibility in medicine (e.g., patient throughput, transitions of care) the team can develop a strategy to neutralize potentially detrimental effects.

There are other team-building techniques that your program may utilize (internally or with other stakeholders in the organization, such as the emergency department or nursing staff). For example, conducting group meetings, perhaps quarterly or semiannually, may benefit collaboration. Annual social gatherings may also contribute to workplace harmony. This setting allows the involved parties to communicate in a relaxed atmosphere. It presents an opportunity for people to connect and build relationships.

Participation in joint initiatives is another effective strategy. For example, the hospitalists may team with the nursing department in the Susan J. Komen race for the cure to raise money for breast cancer. Participation in a Ropes course represents another excellent strategy for team building. This may occur as an internal hospitalist practice activity or as an initiative between the hospitalist practice and another group/community. The goals of this program are to explore group interaction, share problem solving, and develop trust. Anticipated outcomes may include enhancement of teamwork, trust, cooperation, goal setting, decision making, and solidarity.

13 Concluding Thoughts

Hospitalist medicine is the fastest-growing medical specialty in U.S. history. It is no wonder that physician recruitment and retention pose such significant challenges for hospitalist practices. Many and diverse factors contribute to these challenges in addition to their historic growth, and they vary from program to program. After reading this book, it is my hope that the reader has acquired an understanding of them along with the related dynamics of recruitment and retention. Successful strategies can be applied only after gaining an appreciation of the challenges. Readers should appreciate that:

- Familiarizing oneself with physician supply and demand dynamics is a useful start to successful recruitment. Understanding the demographic changes occurring within the medical field in conjunction with the generational expectations of the physician recruitment pool is valuable when your program designs a recruitment and retention strategy. In addition, your hospitalist program can make itself indispensible if it possesses an awareness of the changing roll of both PCP and specialist and creates a tactical plan to address this dynamic.
- Developing a solid pool of candidates from which to choose requires knowledge of the hospitalist marketplace as well as familiarity with various recruitment sources. Successful recruitment and retention of these candidates necessitates that a hospitalist program offer a competitive physician compensation package, a flexible practice model and work schedule (with little to no call), a reasonable daily workload, and hospitalist staff stability. Other factors that will affect your recruitment and/or retention efforts include physician compatibility with the community, practice, and hospital culture as well as spousal and family integration within the community.

Hospitalist Recruitment and Retention: Building a Hospital Medicine Program,
By Kenneth G. Simone
Copyright © 2010 Wiley-Blackwell

- After you have narrowed your candidate list on paper via CV screening, the pre-site interview is a crucial time to begin assessment of the candidate. If the candidate passes this assessment, the site visit will serve as a decisive experience for the physician to evaluate your program. It is essential that the site visit is well choreographed, enabling the physician to obtain objective information about the practice, sponsoring hospital, medical and hospital staff, and community. The site visit is also an opportunity for the spouse and family to learn about the community.

- Identification of *the* right candidate can be very challenging. Physician choice should be based on finding a candidate that has similar values and objectives to your hospitalist program. Once you have identified the ideal candidate, how do you seal the deal? The recruitment initiatives discussed in Chapter 7 were presented to allow your program to attract top candidates. Initiatives such as a sign-on bonus, relocation expense reimbursement, medical school loan repayment, and so on, will make your program competitive from a compensation perspective. It is not enough to attract top candidates; your program must also develop strategies to retain them. The initiatives presented in Chapter 8 will hopefully support retention of your physicians. Tools such as an effective orientation program and mentorship program will benefit your newly hired physicians in this regard.

- An effective practice management strategy will support the success of your program, which will in turn support recruitment and retention of top hospitalist physicians. Practice management strategies should include development of an operational plan (e.g., practice support), delineation of the program's scope of service, and creation of practice policies, procedures, and protocols included in a practice manual. Effective practice management also involves short- and long-term strategic planning for your program. This includes joint planning initiatives with the sponsoring hospital. Strategic planning mandates development of a marketing plan. Attaining your practice management goals can only be accomplished through teamwork and effective hospitalist program leadership.

In closing, physician recruitment and retention is not an easy undertaking. In fact, it may be one of the most difficult challenges that your program faces. Effective recruitment and retention is the assurance of longevity for your hospitalist program. The more creative (and proactive) you can be toward this goal, the greater success you will enjoy. If your program can develop effective strategies to succeed at this task, it will go a long way toward securing the future of your program and that of your sponsoring hospital. Keep in mind that flawless execution is the determining factor in the success of the strategic plan. Finally, let us remember what the illustrious Sir Winston Churchill once said: "However beautiful the strategy, you should occasionally look at the results."

REFERENCES

1. Simone, KG, Dichter, JR. *The Hospitalist Program Management Guide*, 2nd ed. Marblehead, MA: HCPro, 2008.
2. Third Annual AAMC Physician Workforce Research Conference, May 2007. Available at http://AAMC Physician Workforce Research Conference. htm.
3. *The Physician's Perspective: Medical Practice in 2008 Survey*. The Physician's Foundation, Boston, MA, October 2008.
4. *Physician Workforce Policy Guidelines for the United States, 2000–2020: Sixteenth Report*. Washington, DC: U.S. Council on Graduate Medical Education, U.S. Department of Health and Human Services, Health Resources and Services Administration, January 2005.
5. Applicants to U.S. medical schools increase. AAMC press release, November 4, 2003.
6. Jolly, P. Medical school tuition and young physicians' indebtedness. *Health Affairs*, 2005;24(2):527–535.
7. Marston, C. *Motivating the "What's in It for Me" Workforce*. Hoboken, NJ: Wiley, 2007.
8. Society of Hospitalist Medicine 2007–2008 Biennual Survey.
9. Buterakos, J, Taylor, DK. Live chat: use of the Internet as a resident physician recruitment tool. *Journal of the American Medical Association*, 2000;283:2456.
10. *2006 Retention Survey*. American Medical Group Association and Cejka Search.
11. Valancy, J. Recruiting and retaining the right physicians. *Family Practice Management*, 2007;28–33.
12. *2007 Physician Retention Survey*, suppl. ed. Cejka Search.
13. *2008 Review of Physician and CRNA Recruiting Initiatives*. Merritt, Hawkins and Associates.
14. *Today's Hospitalist*, 2008 Compensation and Career Survey Special issue.
15. Gosfield, AG. Stark III: refinement, not revolution (part 2). *Family Practice Management*, April 2008;25–27.

Hospitalist Recruitment and Retention: Building a Hospital Medicine Program,
By Kenneth G. Simone
Copyright © 2010 Wiley-Blackwell

16. Darves, B. Mid-levels make a rocky entrance into hospital medicine. *Today's Hospitalist*, January 2007.

17. Taylor, CA, Taylor, JC, Stoller, JK. Exploring leadership competencies in established and aspiring physician leaders: an interview-based study. *Journal of General Internal Medicine*, June 2008;23(6):748–754. Epub March 8, 2008.

18. Ulrich, D, Smallwood, N. Develop your leadership brand. About.com Human Resources.

19. Bennis, W. *On Becoming a Leader*. Reading, MA: Addison-Wesley, 1989.

20. Manohar, U. *Effective leadership styles*. Buzzle.com.

21. Worth, T. New skills for front-line hospitalists: interviewing candidates. *Today's Hospitalist*, March 2008.

22. Kotter, J. *Leading Change*. Boston: Harvard Business School Press, 1996.

23. Guthrie, MB. Challenges in developing physician leadership. *Frontiers in Health Service Management*, 1999;15:3–28.

24. Fulkerson, W, Jr. *Creating a healthy hospital: the demand for physician executives*. Heathcare Library. Cejka Search.com.

25. Eglé, AG. *Leadership presence*. Buzzle.com, 2008.

26. *A Challenge on Hospitalist Career Satisfaction*. Philadelphia: Society of Hospital Medicine, 2006. Available for download at www.hospitalmedicine. org.

27. Cooper, RA, Stoflet, SJ, Wartman, SA. Perceptions of medical school deans and state medical society executives about physician supply. *Journal of the American Medical Association*, 2003;290:2992–2995.

28. Cooper, RA, Getzen, TE, McKee, HJ, Laud, P. Economic and demographic trends signal an impending physician shortage. *Health Affairs*, 2002;21(1):140–154.

29. Cooper, RA. Medical schools and their applicants. *Health Affairs*, 2003;22(4):71–84.

30. Salsberg, ES, Gaetano, JF. Trends in the physician workforce, 1980–2000. *Health Affairs*, September–October 2002;21:165–173.

31. Dichter, JR, Simone, KG. *Tools and Strategies for an Effective Hospitalist Program*. Marblehead, MA: HCPro, 2006.

32. Measuring hospitalist performance: metrics, reports, and dashboards. Unpublished white paper. Philadelphia: Society of Hospital Medicine, 2006. Available for download at www.hospitalmedicine.org.

33. *Physician Supply and Demand: Projections to 2020*. Washington, DC: U.S. Department of Health and Human Services, Health Resources and Services Administration, Bureau of Health Professions, October 2006.

34. Coile, Jr, RC. 10 Factors affecting the physician shortage of the future— next! *Physician Executive*, September–October 2003.

35. Full, JM. *Physician recruitment strategies for a rural hospital*. ache.org.

36. Westfall, C. Strong physician recruitment and retention. *Physician's News Digest*, January 2004.

37. Cohen, JJ. *Physician Workforce Trends and Expectation*. Association of American Medical Colleges, Washington, DC, December 21, 2006.

38. Pratt, MK. On the wards: hospitalists steadily bolster their ranks. *Boston Business Journal*, March 24, 2006.

39. Lurie, JD, Miller, DP, Lindenauer, PK, Wachter, RM, Sox, HC. The potential size of the hospitalist workforce in the United States. *American Journal of Medicine*, 1999;106(4):441–445.

40. Butchbinder, SB, Wilson, M, Melick, CF, Powe, NR. Estimates of costs of primary care physician turnover. *American Journal of Managed Care*, 1999;5:1431–1438.

41. Glassheim, JW. *Managing your medical practice—without an MBA*. www.uoworks.com, July–August 2004.

42. Physicians try to rein in runaway overhead. *ACP Observer*, March 2004.

43. Cornett, D. Expectations of gen-X recruitment candidates. *Physician's News Digest*, January 2005.

44. Bickel, J, Brown, AJ. Generation X: implications for faculty recruitment and development in academic health centers. *Academic Medicine*, 2005;80(3):205–210.

45. Infante, VD. Millennials: a new generation in the workforce-research. BNET.com, March 2001.

46. Thoreson, B. Designing offices, from boomers to Y. *Business Journal of Milwaukee*, September 21, 2007.

47. Generational challenges: breaking the gen-X code. *Practice Strategies*, Spring 2008.

48. Remer, K, Wilson, J. *Motivating Your Generation X and Y Team Members*. PCPS Firm Practice Center, 2004–2005.

49. Withers, P. Retention strategies that respond to worker values. BNET. com, July 2001.

50. Thilmany, J. Passing on know-how: knowledge retention strategies can keep employees' workplace-acquired wisdom from walking out the door when they retire. BNET.com, June 2008.

INDEX

Academic hospitalist programs, 30, 35–36, 58, 89. *See also* Teaching hospitals
Accountability, 10, 185
Accreditation Council for Graduate Medical Education (ACGME), 17, 30
Added-value benefits, 62, 66
Added-value services, 40–41, 64, 75
Administrative culture, 184
Administrative skills, 41, 76, 78, 89, 96
Administrative systems, 12–13, 15, 24, 27, 40–42, 119, 121, 146, 165–166
Adult-only hospitalist program, 33, 59–60
Advanced practice nurses (APNs), 15–16
Advertising, 46–47, 150
Affiliated hospital, control/hospital governance, 31
Aging population, 2–4, 88
Altruism, organizational, 170, 172
American Academy of Family Physicians (AAFP), 48
American Academy of Pediatricians (AAP), 48
American College of Physicians (ACP), 48
American Medical Association (AMA), 1, 4–5, 12, 18, 21
American Medical Group Association (AMGA), 93
Analytical skills, 126, 128
Antitrust laws, 89–90
Association of American Medical Colleges (AAMC), 1–2, 4, 6, 12, 21
Autonomy, 12, 88, 150, 189–190

Average daily census (ADC), 26, 31, 33–34, 62–63, 65, 149
Average length of stay (ALOS), 31, 37, 65, 67, 69

Baby boomer generation, 18–19, 21
Background check, 106, 119
Behavioral interviewing techniques, 126–128
Behavioral styles, leadership and, 170
Benchmarking, 78–79, 82
Benefits packages, 84, 87, 140
Bennis, Warren, 174
Billing protocol, 75, 99, 153–154
Biostatistics, 67
Board members, roles of, 13, 118
Body language, 123
Bonuses, 7, 61, 83, 85–86, 91, 140, 194
Budgets/budgeting, 145–147
Burnout, 8, 63–64, 91–92, 162, 181, 186, 188
Business skills, 96, 125, 130, 168
Buy-out clause, 141
Bylaws, 138, 150

Call schedule, 32, 34–36, 58–59, 61–65, 94, 97, 103, 140, 188
Candidates:
    assessment of, 123–124
    attraction strategies, 57
    decision-making process, 66, 68
    initial contact with, 104–106
    job description, 41
    local physicians, 50
    pools, identification of, 50–55
    profile development, 121

Hospitalist Recruitment and Retention: Building a Hospital Medicine Program,
By Kenneth G. Simone
Copyright © 2010 Wiley-Blackwell

204 INDEX

Hiring:
    errors, 106
    job offers, 105, 133–134
    mismatch, xii, 39
    personality testing, 133
    protocol, 134–135
Holiday coverage/schedules, 65, 154
Home health services, 153, 190
Hospice services, 190
Hospital(s), *see specific types of hospitals*
    beds, number of, 31–33
    culture, 58, 66–67, 184
    financial health of, 121
    governance, 31
    medical staff credentials committee,
        13
    mission, 30, 67
    performance team, 162
    privileges, 10
    regulation of, 12–14, 138
    size of, 31–33, 105
    subsidies, 29–30, 35, 38, 149
    support from, 58, 69
    systems, 58, 66–67
    teaching status, 29–31
Hospital-dedicated physicians, 9–10
Hospital-employed programs, 85, 87–88
Hospital-hospitalist collaboration, 164
Hospitalist, generally:
    age, gender, and years employed,
        23–25
    community, 190
    education, 26–28
    experienced, 51–52
    initiatives, 156
    leaders, 23–25, 41–42
    local groups, 38, 85, 146
    management companies, 35–36
    marketplace, *see* Hospitalist
        marketplace
    movement, 13–14
    private, 30, 89
    programs, *see* Hospitalist programs
    recruitment pool, *see* Hospitalist
        recruitment pool
    roles of, 37–44
    staffing, 33–34
Hospitalist marketplace:
    affiliated hospital, control/hospital, 31
    coverage schedule, 34–36, 40, 63

    employment model, 29–31
    geographic census regions, 28
    hospital size, 31–33
    hospital teaching status, 29–31
    night call responsibility, 34–36
    practice location, 27–29
    valuation components, 89–90
Hospitalist programs:
    challenges to, 57–71
    growth of, 36
    hospital-owned, 33, 89, 146
    integrated, 94
    popularity of, 57
    responsibilities of, 111
    turnover and, 36
Hospitalist recruitment pool:
    building recruitment network, 45–50
    candidate pool, identification of,
        50–55, 193
Hospital Quality Alliance (HQA), 160

Iacocca, Lee, 171
ICD-9 coding guidelines, 99
IHI, 78, 161
Immigration status, 139, 142
Incentive plans/programs, 61, 73–74,
    79–82, 85, 140
Information sharing, 166
Information technology, 41, 74, 118,
    159–162, 168
Initial contact, 104–106. *See also* First
    impressions
Inpatient management, 10, 15, 39, 88
In-service training, 94
Institute of Medicine (IOM), 17
Insurance industry, 2, 14–15. *See also*
    specific types of insurance
Integrated healthcare delivery team, 43
Integrated hospitalist program with
    hospitalist physicians, 94
Integrated networks, 66
Intensive care/intensive care unit (ICU),
    43, 54, 150
Internal medicine, 24, 26, 44, 88
Internal medicine-pediatric (IM-Ped)
    physicians, 26, 54, 150
International medical school graduates
    (IMGs), 2, 5–6, 17, 54–55, 139, 150
Internet job sites, 47
Interpersonal relationships, 190–192